Developmental Disabilities: A Handbook for Occupational Therapists

The *Occupational Therapy in Health Care* series
Jerry A. Johnson, Editor
Florence S. Cromwell, Editor Emerita

Developmental Disabilities: A Handbook for Occupational Therapists

Jerry A. Johnson
Editor
David A. Ethridge
Co-Editor

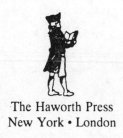

The Haworth Press
New York • London

Developmental Disabilities: A Handbook for Occupational Therapists has also been published as *Occupational Therapy in Health Care*, Volume 6, Numbers 2/3 1989.

The Haworth Press, Inc., 10 Alice Street, Binghamton, NY 13904-1580
EUROSPAN/Haworth, 3 Henrietta Street, London WC2E 8LU England

Library of Congress Cataloging-in-Publication Data

Developmental disabilities : a handbook for occupational therapists / Jerry A. Johnson, editor ;
David A. Ethridge, co-editor.
p. cm.
Has also been published as : Occupational therapy in health care, v. 6, no. 2/3.
Includes bibliographical references.
ISBN 0-86656-959-6
1. Developmentally disabled—Rehabilitation. 2. Occupational therapy. I. Johnson, Jerry A.
II. Ethridge, David A. [DNLM: 1. Autism—rehabilitation. 2. Cerebral Palsy—rehabilitation. 3.
Epilepsy—rehabilitation. 4. Mental Retardation—rehabilitation. 5. Occupational Therapy, W1
OC601H
RC570.2.D48   1989
616.8—dc20
DNLM/DLC
for Library of Congress   89-20012
                                                                                               CIP

Developmental Disabilities: A Handbook for Occupational Therapists

CONTENTS

BOOK REVIEWS

ABOUT THE EDITORS

Jerry A. Johnson, MBA, EdD, OTR, FAOTA, is President of Context, Inc., and Editor of *Occupational Therapy in Health Care*. She was Founder, Professor, and Director of the Occupational Therapy Department at Boston University (1963-1971), and more recently was Professor and Elias Michael Director of Occupational Therapy at Washington University in St. Louis. She served as President of the American Occupational Therapy Association for over five years and is a recipient of both The Eleanor Clarke Slagle Lectureship and the Award of Merit, AOTA's two highest awards. She serves as a national and international lecturer and consultant.

David A. Ethridge, PhD, OTR, FAOTA, is Director of Oakdale Regional Center, a large state facility in Lapeer, Michigan for mentally retarded people. Dr. Ethridge also serves as an appointee of AOTA and the Accreditation Council and has been elected to serve as President of the Council for 1989. Dr. Ethridge has published extensively in the areas of research and mental health and serves as a consultant to various mental health programs in several states. He has recently been appointed by the World Federation of Occupational Therapists to serve as an expert advisor to the World Health Organization.

Developmental Disabilities:
A Handbook
for Occupational Therapists

FROM THE EDITOR

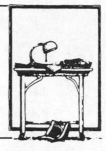

This volume represents a significant accomplishment in bringing together many articles concerned with the broad range of individuals with developmental disabilities and the variety of services that are needed to address the multiple problems confronted by individuals with development disabilities handicaps and by their families. Given the scope of this field, this collection is by no means complete, or even comprehensive, but it docs provide broad coverage of the spectrum of problems confronted by patients and the many kinds of occupational therapy services these individuals need.

David Ethridge, as Co-Editor, has provided the primary source of expertise in this volume. He and the contributing authors deserve recognition and appreciation for their commitment, perseverance, and contributions to this volume on developmental disabilities. I am grateful to each of them and hope that these papers will make a significant contribution to those occupational therapists who work with persons having developmental disabilities.

Jerry A. Johnson
Editor

1

FROM THE CO-EDITOR

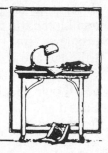

As an occupational therapist privileged to be appointed by the American Occupational Therapy Association to sit as one of their representatives on the Accreditation Council on Services for People with Developmental Disabilities (ACDD) I have been frequently asked for assistance in identifying programs or agencies which exemplify quality occupational therapy practice in the field of developmental disabilities. It is always difficult to answer such queries. Likewise, we have frequently been asked for references to current literature which would assist new therapists to acclimate to caseloads of persons with developmental disabilities. There continues to be a severe paucity of professional literature dealing with occupational therapy and developmental disabilities.

This volume is an attempt to address both questions; that of identifying programs and therapists involved in quality practice and to add to the professional literature in the field of occupational therapy and developmental disabilities. No single volume can ever contain all the subjects desired but an attempt has been made to cover the major disability groupings generally encompassed in the broad term, developmental disabilities: autism, cerebral palsy, epilepsy and mental retardation. Papers were solicited which represented both institutional and community service programs; dealt with both children and adults; and ranged from mild to severe levels of impairment.

The initial three articles deal with specific approaches to specific developmental disabilities; Bloomer and Rose on autism, Kibele and Llorens on cerebral palsy, and Clerico on epilepsy. Institutional programs for persons with mental retardation are covered by Ethridge and colleagues, Stratton, Lust and colleagues and Lewin. Community based programs are described by Case-Smith, Herrick and Lowe, Jackson and colleagues, and Stout and colleagues. Schaaf and Gitlen looks at early intervention tool, Transon and colleagues at grip strength and dexterity and finally Shaperman and Lewis remind us of the importance of program evaluation.

Many of the contributors to this volume are first-time authors and it has been particularly gratifying to work with them to bring their ideas and manuscripts to final form. It is through such seeking out of individuals willing to contribute their time and energies that expansion of our literature is accomplished. My thanks to them for their many, many hours of hard work and their patience in the lengthy review and rewrite process. My thanks also to the reviewers who contributed many good ideas to facilitate revisions when needed. It is our hope that this series of articles will prove useful to our field and will encourage more therapists to express their unique and valuable experiences so that we may all continue to learn.

David A. Ethridge
Co-Editor

Frames of Reference:
Guiding Treatment for Children
with Autism

MaryAnn L. Bloomer, OTR/L
Catherine C. Rose, OTR/L

SUMMARY. Children with autism vary greatly in their individual learning styles, their problem areas, and their response to treatment. Since children with this diagnosis present a relatively unique clinical picture, innovative approaches to treatment are required. The purpose of this paper is to encourage therapists to employ a variety of treatment techniques according to the traditional frames of reference described in the occupational therapy literature (Tiffany, 1983; Matsutsuyu, 1983; Ayres, 1979; Pedretti and Pasquelli-Estrada, 1985). These include the following approaches: developmental, occupational behavior, sensory integrative, acquisitional, biomechanical, rehabilitative, and psychoanalytic. Each frame of reference will be described in terms of its theoretical base, state of dysfunction, and focus of intervention in order to assist the therapist in developing a structured approach in initiating treatment. In addition, a theoretical case study will be presented and each frame of reference applied with an emphasis on principles for treatment and sample long and

---

MaryAnn Bloomer received her BS in occupational therapy from Washington University in 1985 and a BS in education and psychology from Webster University Community Pediatric Services. Catherine Rose graduated with distinction from the Washington University Program in Occupational Therapy in 1987. She is presently a staff therapist with Washington University Community Pediatric Services, 4567 Scott Avenue, St. Louis, MO 63110.

The authors would like to thank Dr. Margo Holm for her articulate presentation to the profession of the clinical definitions and uses of frames of reference with the developmentally disabled population (Project for Independent Living, American Occupational Therapy Association, 1986). We would also like to extend our appreciation to the Program in Occupational Therapy at Washington University for its support in the preparation of this manuscript.

5

short term goals. Suggestions will also be provided for establishing a therapeutic environment for children with autism.

INTRODUCTION

Providing occupational therapy for children with autism presents a challenge to the clinician. Each child presents a different clinical picture. The response to therapeutic techniques may vary greatly from one child to the next. Therefore, the occupational therapist must try a variety of treatment approaches to help facilitate the child's maximum skill development. When one approach proves to be ineffective or insufficient, the therapist should consider trying new techniques. By using the frames of reference as a treatment guide, the therapist is provided with concepts, definitions, statements, descriptions and plans of action. This approach offers structure to the task of treating children with a complex pervasive disorder.

ORDERING CONCEPTUAL INFORMATION

Theories, frames of reference, and activities provide the basis for planning and implementing occupational therapy interventions. According to Holm (1986), it is important to understand the relationship of these constructs when developing treatment plans for individuals with developmental disabilities. Holm defines these terms as follows:

1. *Theories* consist of concepts, definitions, statements, and postulates that describe the relationship among concepts. A theory describes phenomena so as to explain or predict. Examples of theories might include the theory of operant conditioning and theories of growth and development. A theory is universal in scope. Teachers, counselors, physical therapists, and other team members may use these theories, as do occupational therapists.
2. A *frame of reference* is derived from a theory. In addition to

concepts and definitions, it also includes a guide for action that is specific to a practitioner's domain. Intervention strategies are included to facilitate change. For example, a teacher and an occupational therapist may both be working from a developmental theory base, but their intervention strategies will be quite different because of their specific areas of concentration.

3. *Activities* are tasks, techniques, projects, or processes designed to assist the child in reaching a goal. Without a frame of reference and theoretical base, the activity may or may not be therapeutic (Holm, 1986).

Table 1 summarizes the following frames of reference for occupational therapy intervention: developmental, occupational behavior, sensory integrative, acquisitional, biomechanical, rehabilitative, and psychoanalytic. Each frame of reference is described in terms of its theoretical base, state of dysfunction, and focus of intervention.

CHOOSING A FRAME OF REFERENCE

According to Holm (1986), many factors contribute to the therapist's decision to utilize a particular frame of reference. These may include the child's problem area, goal and allotted time for treatment, philosophy of the program, or the knowledge and skills of the therapist. The therapist will need to take into account the child's disability, age, problem areas, and personal preference when choosing a treatment approach. The opinion of the parent will also be a factor to consider.

The therapy goals and the time line in which the therapist is working influence the choice of a frame of reference. The developmental, occupational behavior, sensory integrative and biomechanical approaches all require long term treatment intervention for the sequential development of skills. When the treatment time line is limited, the therapist may choose to utilize the acquisitional or the rehabilitative approach.

The program philosophy and the knowledge base of the therapist are other determining factors when considering a treatment ap-

TABLE 1. Occupational Therapy Frames of Reference

Theoretical Frame of Reference	Theoretical Frame of Reference
---------------------	---------------
Acquisitional	Biomechanical

Theoretical base: Humans learn by interacting with a reinforcing environment through practice and repetition.	Theoretical base: Humans can develop physical sub-skills based on range of motion, strength and endurance.
State of Dysfunction: Unable to perform the skills needed for a given environment and/or to generalize skills to new conditions.	State of Dysfunction: Unable to perform the physical sub-skills necessary for activities of daily living such as range of motion, strength and endurance.
Focus of Intervention: Provide opportunities to practice specific skills with appropriate reinforcement in familiar and unfamiliar environments.	Focus of Intervention: Increase range of motion, strength and endurance through graded activities.
Evaluation: Skills check list.	Evaluation: Range of motion (goniometry) Manual muscle test Pinch/grip strength Endurance testing Position and body mechanics.
Establishment of Goals: STO: Acquire skills through practice in clinical setting LTO: Acquire skills that can be generalized to community environment.	Establishment of Goals: STO: Perform physical subskills in clinical setting. LTO: Perform physical subskills as needed for independent living skills.

proach. Certain treatment programs or school settings have a specific philosophy from which all professionals work, e.g., developmental, acquisitional, or rehabilitation. The therapist may use one frame of reference because of personal experience and knowledge. Likewise, a therapist may elect not to use a certain approach be-

Theoretical Frame of Reference	Theoretical Frame Of Reference
-----------------	-----------------------
Developmental	Occupational Behavior
Theoretical base: Humans develop tasks and roles according to a predictable sequence.	Theoretical base: Humans are biological, psycho-social, and cultural beings who spontaneously explore and master their environment.
State of Dysfunction: Unable to perform physical and daily living skills in an age appropriate manner.	State of Dysfunction: Unable to develop role requirements in the areas of work, play, self care.
Focus of Intervention: Establish baseline level of performance and provide activities along the developmental continuum.	Focus of Intervention: Acquire and perform skills of work, play and self care.
Evaluation: Developmental assessment.	Evaluation: History taking Role assessment Inventory of activities of daily living, play skills Work assessment
Establishment of Goals: STO: Perform age appropriate skills in the clinical setting. LTO: Perform age appropriate skills in the community environment.	Establishment of Goals: STO: Develop life skills and personal interest while in the clinical setting. LTO: Develop life skills and personal interests that can be maintained in the community environment.

cause he or she lacks the skill development and credentials, e.g., sensory integration or neurodevelopmental treatment certifications.

It should be noted that more than one frame of reference may be used at the same time to work on the presenting problem areas provided they are not conflicting. Also, when progress levels off with one treatment approach, the therapist may wish to initiate another approach to best facilitate the child's maximum skill development.

TABLE 1 (continued)

Theoretical Frame Of Reference	Theoretical Frame Of Reference
--------------------------	---------------
Sensory Integration	Rehabilitation

Theoretical base: Humans organize sensory input through the central nervous system in order to respond to the environment in a meaningful way.	Theoretical base: Humans are capable of adapting to their limitations by learning new methods of performing through compensation or adaptive aids.
State of Dysfunction: Unable to respond appropriately to sensory input.	State of Dysfunction: Unable to demonstrate skills and behaviors necessary for independent functioning.
Focus of Intervention: Provide controlled sensory input through sensory motor activities and sensory integration techniques to ellicit an adaptive response	Focus of Intervention: Develop compensation techniques through patient education and training in environmental adaptations.
Evaluation: SI tests Sensorimotor history	Evaluation: Life skills evaluation Needs assessment
Establishment of Goals: STO: Exhibit an adaptive response to sensory input in the clinical setting. LTO: Exhibit an adaptive response to sensory input in the community environment.	Establishment of Goals: STO: Perform life skills in clinical setting using compensatory techniques. LTO: Perform life skills in community environment using compensatory techniques.

LITERATURE REVIEW OF AUTISM

Autism was first described by Leo Kanner in 1943. Since that time, several researchers have attempted to identify the etiological factors and characteristics of the condition (Rutter, 1978; Ornitz and Ritvo; 1976, Kolvin, 1971). The Diagnostic and Statistical

Theoretical
Frame Of Reference

Psychoanalytic

Theoretical base:
Human behavior is based on unconscious
biological drives. These drives become
conscious, are resolved and intrapsychic
development continues.

State of Dysfunction:
Unable to control unconscious
conflict which interferes with intrapersonal
and interpersonal development.

Focus of Intervention:
Uncover unconscious conflicts
which interfere with performance
through expressive therapy.

Evaluation:
Projective art techniques
Role play
Stress Inventory

Establishment of Goals:
STO: Project unconscious conflict
through expressive media in
the clinical setting.
LTO: Resolve unconscious conflict
for independent functioning
in the community
environment.

Manual of Mental Disorders (DSM III, 1980) lists the following
criteria for the diagnosis of infantile autism:

A. onset before 30 months of age;
B. pervasive lack of responsiveness to other people;
C. gross deficits in language development;
D. peculiar speech patterns such as immediate and delayed
   echolalia, metaphorical language, pronominal reversal (if
   speech is present);
E. bizarre responses to various aspects of the environment, e.g.,

resistance to change, peculiar interest in or attachments to animate or inanimate objects; and
F. an absence of delusions, hallucinations, loosening of associations, and incoherence, as in schizophrenia.

Other factors that may accompany autism often include perceptual and sensory processing disturbances, unusual motility patterns, and mental retardation (Ramm, 1983). Wing (1976) summarizes evidence documenting the presence of autism in four or five of every 10,000 children. Boys are affected up to four times as often as girls (Wing, 1976). Autism occurs throughout the world and in children from all backgrounds.

To date, the exact cause of autism is unknown. A review of the literature on autism points to three main theoretical categories regarding the etiology of the disease (Wolkowicz, Fish, Schaffer, 1977): (1) the psychodynamically oriented theories, (2) the organic-experiential interaction theories, and (3) the organic theories. The psychodynamic theories assume that the autistic child is born physically normal, and that psychotic behavior develops later on because of maternal disinterest and lack of affection. The universality of such findings has been questioned (Margolies, 1977).

The organic-experiential interaction theories combine the viewpoints of both the psychodynamic and organic theories. These theories can be divided into two categories: (a) those which emphasize an unhealthy mother-child relationship while allowing for vulnerability in the child, and (b) those which stress deviation in the child for which the mother does not compensate (Wolkowicz, Fish, Schaffer, 1977). These theories propose that the various hereditary and biological factors are present, but that the parents are still at least partially responsible for influencing the emergence of the disorder.

Today there is general agreement among most researchers that autism is caused by organic brain pathology (Schanzenbacher, 1985). Schlopler (1965) noted that children with autism respond abnormally to sensory stimulation, while Rimland (1964) hypothesized that the brain stem reticular formation somehow relates to the disorder. Both of these theories suggest a neuropathophysiologic basis for the etiology of autism. Studies pursuing this line of investigation may be classified as those proposing (a) a sensory processing disturbance, (b) aberrant cerebral specializations, and (c) atypical memory, arousal, and attentional mechanisms (Clark, 1983). In addition, Nelson (1984) discusses evidence indicating that children with autism have a disorder in the modulation between sensory input and motor output, which may explain their inconsistent motor responses.

A number of well executed studies have suggested that perceptual disturbances may contribute to the etiology of autism (Clark, 1983). Many of these neurophysiological findings point strongly to the presence of a vestibular disorder in autism. When studying the effects of vestibular stimulation on rapid eye movement (REM) sleep, Ornitz and colleagues (1973) found that children with autism, unlike the control group, do not demonstrate an increase in eye movement burst duration as a result of vestibular stimulation. These authors speculated that the disturbances in modulation and registration of sensory input associated with autism may be linked to a vestibular disorder. Other studies have shown that children with autism have diminished pose rotary nystagmus after their vestibular system is stimulated by spinning (Piggot, 1979). The nystagmus is only inhibited when the child is spun in a lighted room; in a dark room, the child with autism has a normal amount of post rotary nystagmus. This finding may also indicate a defect in the integration of visual and vestibular stimulation.

Other research has implied that children with autism have disturbances in auditory processing. Student and Sohmer (1978) used auditory nerve and brain stem evoked responses to study the auditory processing of children with autistic traits. Results indicated significantly different evoked responses when comparing the control group to the children with autistic traits. The type of waves found in children with autism were characterized by prolonged latencies indicting immaturity, which could possibly lead to distorted images of the outside world.

Over the last 15 years, research has indicated abnormal hemispheric dominance patterns in autism. DeLong (1978) found that 13 out of 17 children meeting many of the criteria for autism demonstrated enlargement of the left ventricular system, especially the left temporal horns. These anatomical malformations were in the area of the limbic system. Hier et al., (1979) reported that the computerized tomography (CT) scans of 9 out of 16 autistic children demonstrated reversed symmetry in the posterior language region, which may contribute to the limited language acquisition in children with autism. Blastock (1978) noted that children with autism seem to prefer musical over verbal input, suggesting that they may prefer processing information in the right rather than the left hemisphere. Lastly children with autism seem to show a nongenetically related higher incidence of left-handedness, also indicating left hemisphere dysfunction (Boucher, 1977; Colby and Parkinson, 1977).

Other studies have suggested that disturbances in memory and attentional mechanisms may contribute to the etiology of autism. The possible defects in the limbic system previously mentioned (DeLong, 1978) seem to implicate memory disturbances in children with autism. Hutt et al., (1965) identified the child with autism as being physiologically over-stimulated and therefore unable to process sensory input. The authors hypothesize that the repetitive stimulation often noted may serve as an arousal-reducing function. According to Ramm (1983), children with autism receive inadequate sensory stimulation and therefore commonly seek it through atypical motility patterns. The observed hypersensitivity or hyposensitivity to stimuli may be due to a defect in the ability to selectively attend to a task (Grandin, 1984). Kootz et al., (1982) suggest that children with autism avoid stimulation and resort to self-stimulating behaviors to "flood sensory receptors and insist on an unchanging environment."

In summary, it appears that neurophysiological factors may contribute to the etiology of autism. There is strong evidence that dysfunction of the sensory systems, limbic system, arousal mechanisms, as well as aberrant cerebral lateralization may contribute to the emergence of the disorder.

REVIEW OF THE OCCUPATIONAL THERAPY LITERATURE

According to Levine (1981), only eight articles in the *American Journal of Occupational Therapy* from 1947-1981 mention autism, and few additions have been made since that time. Although the use of milieu therapy, behavior modification, play facilitation, and crafts have been described in the occupational therapy literature, sensory integrative therapy appears to be the most frequently mentioned treatment for children with autism. The neurophysiological theories of etiology have formed the basis for much of the occupational therapy research regarding the sensory integrative treatment of children with autism.

Jean Ayres, the founder of sensory integrative therapy, did much of her research with the learning disabled population; however, applications are now being made to children with autism. In *Sensory Integration and the Child* (1979), Ayres identifies three aspects of poor sensory processing that are noted in the child with autism: (1) sensory input is not being "registered" correctly in the child's brain, resulting in hypoactivity and hyperactivity to stimulation; (2) the child may not modulate sensory input well, especially vestibular and tactile sensations; and (3) brain dysfunction causes the child to have little interest in performing constructive and purposeful activities. Activities involving movement experiences and deep touch sensations are hypothesized by Ayres to help the child with autism create more adaptive responses to the environment.

In one study, Ayres and Heskett (1972) used tactile and vestibular stimulation with a seven year old girl with autism for a six month treatment period. Post treatment testing showed considerable gains in perceptual-motor skills, auditory-language functions, and reading. Likewise, Wolkowicz, Fish and Schaffer (1977) found that the use of sensory integrative therapy was beneficial to four children with autism in increasing sensory integrative functioning and improving behavioral and social skills after a four month treatment period.

Ayres and Tickle (1980) found that children with autism who tend to be hyper-responsive to touch and vestibular stimulation respond better to sensory integrative therapy than those who fail to orient to sensory input. All of these studies appear to indicate the possibility that at least some children with autism benefit from sensory integrative therapy (Clark, 1983).

Results have not been published in the occupational therapy literature which contradict the use of sensory integration for children with autism. However, in one study (Reilly, Nelson, Bundy, 1983), the spontaneous vocalizations of 18 children with autism were compared after sensory integrative therapy and traditional fine motor activities. Contrary to expectations, fine motor, rather than sensorimotor activities, elicited significantly more variety of speech, greater average length of utterances, and less echolalic speech.

The occupational therapy literature also describes the use of behavior modification, play facilitation, crafts, and music therapy in treating children with autism. In *The Developmental Therapist* (1971), Kent describes the use of behavior therapy in treatment of children with pervasive disorders and with children who display limited appropriate behaviors. She suggests that occupational therapy can be utilized to modify behavior through the use of positive reinforcers. Wehman and Abramson (1976) reviewed three theories of play and described each in terms of their applicability to exceptional children. They reported that play activities can be used effectively to mediate the development of adaptive behavior in children with behavioral deficits.

In two articles (1960 and 1961), Weston discussed the use of crafts for children with autism, focusing on the features of craft activities in relation to behavioral problems. He presented selection criteria for using craft activities therapeutically to help facilitate "personality growth" for children with the disorder. Lastly, Farmer (1963) described the use of a musical activity program with four girls diagnosed with "childhood schizophrenia," explaining that the girls learned from the program and derived satisfaction and enjoyment.

Although many treatment theories exist, little conclusive evidence is available upon which to base occupational therapy treatment with the autistic population. Furthermore, each child with autism responds to therapy in a different way, so the therapist may need to try a variety of approaches to help maximize the child's skill development.

CASE STUDY EXAMPLE

This theoretical case study is presented to illustrate the use of the frames of reference outlined in this paper. Specific skill deficits and behavioral characteristics of children with autism are included.

Brian is a 9-year-old male with a primary diagnosis of infantile autism. When encouraged, he is able to speak intelligibly with a vocabulary of 50 words. He does not initiate conversation with peers or adults. He does not play cooperatively with peers. Spontaneous interaction with toys is nonpurposeful and self-stimulatory. Brian has a peculiar interest in preferred inanimate objects upon which he fixates for extended periods of time.

In occupational therapy, Brian avoids a variety of tactile sensations and movement experiences. When placed on moving equipment, he cries. Fine and gross motor skills are within the 3-1/2 to 4-year level. Muscle tone is low. Overall strength and endurance are decreased for age level expectations. Brian is easily distracted and his decreased attention span interferes with his ability to attend to a toy or activity for longer than 30 seconds. Under direct supervision and with physical assistance, he is able to interact appropriately with toys and in activities that are at the 3-4 year level.

One of Brian's problems, the inability to independently play with toys in a meaningful way, will be utilized to illustrate the use of the frames of reference for developing treatment techniques. This problem was selected for illustration because of its implication in a child's interaction with his environment. A child's interaction with toys is important for the following reasons: a)it provides opportunities for increased interaction with peers and caregivers; b)it allows for increased opportunities to develop fine/gross motor and intellectual skills; and c)it provides the child with opportunities to actively explore his physical environment.

Table 2 outlines the use of each frame for possible remediation of this particular problem.

ESTABLISHING A THERAPEUTIC ENVIRONMENT FOR CHILDREN WITH AUTISM

The following general suggestions are intended to assist the therapist in establishing a therapeutic environment. They do not provide specific suggestions for individual problems or address a particular

TABLE 2. Case Study of Brian

Theoretical Frame of Reference Developmental	Theoretical Frame of Reference Occupational Behavior
Assumed Cause for Problem: Brian cannot independently play with a toy because he is developmentally delayed in the acquisition of age appropriate play skills.	Assumed Cause for Problem: Brian cannot independently play with a toy because he has not developed the self care, work, and play skills required for his role as a child and a student.
Principle for Treatment: Participation in play activities progressing along the developmental continuum will result in more independent play at an age-appropriate level.	Principle for Treatment: Utilizing a variety of self-care, school, and play activities in his role as a child will give Brian practice in developing appropriate play skills and result in more independent play.
Short-Term Goal: By January 1, Brian will play with a toy (4 year level) with only verbal cues and no physical assistance.	Short-Term Goal: By January 1, Brian will play with a classroom toy with only verbal cues from a therapist.
Long-Term Goal: By June 1, Brian will demonstrate the ability to play independently with a given toy, game, or piece of equipment for a three minute time period.	Long-Term Goal: By June 1, Brian will demonstrate the ability to play independently with a given toy, game or piece of equipment for a three minute time period.

frame of reference. The intention is to assist the therapist in developing a structured environment, which is necessary when initiating treatment for children with autism.

1. Review all available records and note all important information including previous illness, medications, medical reports, treatment records, and level of progress achieved. Keep notations in a file for quick reference.

Theoretical Frame of Reference	Theoretical Frame of Reference
Sensory Integration	Acquisitional

Assumed Cause for Problem:
Brian cannot correclty "register" sensory input thus he has little interest in performing purposeful play activities.

Assumed Cause for Problem:
Brian cannot play independently with a toy because he has not acquired the necessary cognitive and motor skills.

Principle for Treatment:
Participation in activities which involve controlled sensory input will improve Brian's abillity to respond adaptively to his environment, and result in an increased ability to play independently.

Principle for Treatment:
Repetition and practice in play skills of graded difficulty will improve Brian's ability to play independently.

Short-Term Goal:
By January 1, Brian will initiate play on one piece of equipment in the occupational therapy clinic designed to provide tactile stimulation.

Short-Term Goal:
By January 1, Brian will be able to string four 1" beads with only verbal cues from the therapist.

Long-Term Goal:
By June 1, Brian will demonstrate the ability to play independently with a given toy, game, or piece of equipment for a three minute time period.

Long-Term Goal:
By June 1, Brian will demonstrate the ability to play independently with a given toy, game, or piece of equipment for a three minute time period.

2. Consult with parents, caregivers and teachers to discuss the child's history, habits, behavior patterns, preferences, non-preferred activities, motivators, and child's mode of communication (request examples).
3. Discuss anticipated goals. What does the parent/teacher expect this child to achieve in occupational therapy?
4. Observe the child 2-3 times in different settings (if possible). Inquire if the behavior demonstrated is typical.
5. Determine the teacher's and staff's most effective methods of interaction with the child.

TABLE 2 (continued)

Theoretical Frame of Reference Biomechanical	Theoretical Frame of Reference Rehabilitation
Assumed Cause for Problem: Brian has not developed independent play skills because of this poor upper extremity strength and endurance.	Assumed Cause for Problem: Brian is unable to adapt to his environment therefore the environment must be adapted for him so that he is able to play independently.
Principle for Treatment: Participation in activities to increase upper extremity strength and endurance will improve Brian's fine motor development and result in more independent play.	Principle for Treatment: By adapting the environment to decrease the external distractions, Brian will be able to attend to a toy and consequently play independently.
Short-Term Goal: By January 1, Brian will improve his grip and pinch strength by five pounds each.	Short-Term Goal: By January 1, Brian will play independently with a toy for one minute in a small treatment room with only a table, the toy, and the therapist.
Long-Term Goal: By June 1, Brian will demonstrate the ability to play independently with a given toy, game, or piece of equipment for a three minute time period.	Long-Term Goal: By June 1, Brian will demonstrate the ability to play independently with a given toy, game, or piece of equipment for a three minute time period.

6. Participate with the child in the classroom setting 2-3 times in order to help the child familiarize himself/herself with the therapist.

7. Evaluate the child using clinical observations, informal assessment tools (checklists), or formal tests (when applicable).

8. Select realistic occupational therapy goals in conjunction

Theoretical
Frame of Reference

Psychoanalytic

Assumed Cause for Problem:
Brian is unable to play independently because he is not able to
control biological drives or
resolve intrapsychic conflicts.

Principle for Treatment:
Through projective means, Brian
will reveal unconscious conflicts
which interfere with performance
in independent play skills.

Short-Term Goal:
By January 1, Brian will express
his frustrations in a finger painting
activity under the supervision of
the therapist.

Long-Term Goal:
By June 1, Brian will demonstrate
the ability to play independently
with a given toy, game, or piece of
equipment for a three minute time
period.

with the parent's and teacher's suggestions. Select the appropriate frame of reference to achieve these goals.

9. Develop a treatment routine for each child. Be as consistent
as possible, especially in the familiarization stage.

10. Introduce equipment in gradual steps, especially if the child
has an aversive reaction to a particular sensation. Grade the
activity from verbal introduction to increased physical participation.

11. Keep the physical aspects of the treatment environment con-

sistent, i.e., regular treatment time, location and position of the table and equipment.

12. Clear the work area of all other materials; remove as many distractions as possible. Place only 1-2 objects in front of the child at a time. Use hand over hand assistance if required. Select an appropriate sized table or mat depending on the child's age, ability and tolerance.

13. Use oneself as a therapeutic tool. Place one's body in the most advantageous position, i.e., some children will benefit from having visual feedback. Others perform better when the therapist gives hand overhand assistance and provides physical clues.

14. Use a low modulated voice. Talk with the child about the activity. Praise and encouragement are important despite the child's inability to provide consistent verbal feedback.

15. Break down the tasks and verbalize the steps as the child progresses through the activity. Reduce verbal prompts as the child becomes more independent.

16. Alternate between preferred and more challenging (or stressful) activities. Treatment sessions should conclude with a pleasant preferred task.

17. Use a variety of calming techniques to determine the most effective methods. These preferred techniques may be useful in time of agitation or following stressful activities.

18. Modify the length of the treatment session depending on the child's tolerance level and abilities.

19. Keep detailed daily progress notes describing the goals addressed, the child's response, his performance level, behavior, and the teacher's remarks.

20. Anticipate a longer than average adjustment period, frequent lapses in abilities, behavior changes due to illnesses or absences, and gradual or fluctuating progress.

21. Maintain open communication with parents and staff who can give daily feedback. Use a log to communicate with home if necessary. Work as a team member reinforcing mutual goals.

NEED FOR THEORETICAL RESEARCH
WITH THE AUTISTIC POPULATION

The effectiveness of the given frames of reference and suggested treatment techniques have not been empirically supported. According to Ottenbacher and York (1984), "the overall validation of therapeutic programs employed with particular patient populations can only occur through the accumulation of evidence in support of a particular theoretical orientation." In most instances, the development of such a body of knowledge requires the use of traditional group comparison research, which involves assembling a large number of subjects and randomly assigning them to experimental and control groups. Such research is often difficult when the population of interest consists of heterogeneous, widely dispersed individuals, as is the case for children with autism. In such cases, an alternate research method may need to be utilized, such as single-subject research designs.

As clinicians, we must be not only concerned with quantitatively testing theory-derived hypotheses, but we must also demonstrate the validity of specific treatment techniques as applied to individual patients in a wide variety of environments. Single subject research is an effective way of documenting patient progress while also establishing therapeutic accountability in a systematic and objective manner (Ottenbacher and York, 1984; Campbell, 1988). In addition, this method allows the therapist flexibility to make changes when a given treatment protocol is not maximally beneficial. The researcher also has the option of grouping treatment results to assess the overall effectiveness of occupational therapy programming. Such a research design may prove to be well suited for studying the effects of treatment for children with autism. Furthermore, the insights gained may assist the researcher in developing theoretical hypotheses for further experimental research.

In closing, the authors would like to encourage occupational therapists to engage in both theory-based empirical research (when possible) and single-subject research designs that will ultimately provide the necessary knowledge and theoretical foundation for developing appropriate treatment interventions for children with autism.

REFERENCES

American Psychiatric Association. (1980). *Diagnostic and statistical manual of mental disorders* (3rd ed.). Washington, DC: Author.

Ayres, A. J. (1979). *Sensory integration and the child.* Los Angeles: Western Psychological Services.

Ayres, A. J., & Heskett, W.M. (1972). Sensory integrative dysfunction in a young girl. *J. of Autism Child Schizophr, 2*(2), 174-181.

Ayres, A. J., & Tickle, L.S. (1980). Hyperresponsivity to touch and vestibular stimuli as a predictor of positive response to sensory integration procedures by autistic children. *Am J Occup Ther, 34*(6), 375-381.

Blastock, E.G. (1978). Cerebral asymmetry and the development of early infantile autism. *J Autism Child Schizophr, 8*, 339-353.

Boucher, J. (1977). Hand preference in autistic children and their parents. *J Autism Child Schizophr, 7*, 177-187.

Campbell, P.H. (1988). Using a single-subject research design to evaluate the effectiveness of treatment. *Am J Occup Ther, 42*(1), 732-738.

Clark, F. (1983). Research on the neuropathophysiology of autism and its implications for occupational therapy. *Occup Ther J of Research, 3*(1), 3-22.

Colby, K.M., & Parkinson, C. (1977). Handedness in autistic children. *J Autism Child Schizophr, 6*, 157-162.

De Long, G.R. (1978). A neurophysiological interpretation of infantile autism. In M. Rutter & Shopler (Eds.), *Autism: A reappraisal of concepts and treatment.* New York: Plenum.

Farmer, R. (1963). A musical activities program with young psychotic girls. *Am J Occup Ther, 17*, 116-119.

Grandin, T. (1984). My experience as an autistic child and review of selected literature. *J Orthomol Psychiatry, 13*(3), 144-174.

Hier, D., LeMay, M., & Rosenberger, P. (1979). Autism and unfavorable left-right asymmetries of the brain. *J Autism Dev Disord, 9*, 153-159.

Holm, M. (1986). Frames of reference: guides for action, occupational therapist. In H. Schmidt (Ed.), *Project for Independent Living in Occupational Therapy.* Rockville, Maryland: American Occupational Therapy Association, pp. 69-78.

Hutt, S.J., Hutt, C., Lee, D., & Ounsted, C. (1965). A behavioral and electroencephalographic study of autistic children. *Journal of Psychiatric Research, 3*, 181-197.

Kent, C. (1971). Psychosocial development: Function and dysfunction. In B. Banus (Ed.), *The developmental therapist-a prototype of the pediatric occupational therapist* (pp. 213-275). Thorofare, NY: Slack.

Kolvin, I. (1971). Psychoses in childhood-A comparative study. In M. Rutter (Ed.), *Infantile autism: Concepts, characteristics, and treatment.* London: Churchill Livingstone.

Kootz, J.P., Marinelli, B., & Cohen, D.J. (1982). Modulation of response to environmental stimulation in autistic children. *J Autism Dev Disord*, *12*, 185-192.

Levine, C.R. (1981). *Survey of assessment and treatment of autistic children in occupational therapy*. Unpublished master's thesis, Washington University, St. Louis, MO.

Margolies, P.J. (1977). Behavioral approaches to the treatment of early infantile autism: A review. *Psychol Bull*, *84*(2), 249-264.

Matsutsuyu, J. (1983). Occupational behavior approaches. In H.L. Hopkins & H.D. Smith (Eds.), *Willard and Spackman's occupation therapy* (6th ed.) (pp. 129-134). Philadelphia, PA: J.B. Lippincott.

Nelson, V. (1984). *Children with autism and other pervasive disorders of development and behavior*. Thorofare, NJ: Slack.

Ornitz, E.M., Forsythe, A.B., & de la Pena, A. (1973). The effect of vestibular and auditory stimulation in the rapid eye movements of REM sleep in normal and autistic children. *Arch Gen Psychiatry*, *29*, 786-791.

Ornitz, E.M., & Ritvo, E.R. (1976). The syndrome of autism: A critical review. *Am J Psychiatry*, *133*, 609-621.

Ottenbacher, K., & York, J. (1984). Strategies for evaluating clinical change: Implications for practice and research. *Am J Occup Ther*, *38*(10), 647-659.

Pedretti, L., & Pasquelli-Estrada, S. (1985). *Foundations for treatment of physical occupational therapy practice skills for physical dysfunction* (2nd ed.). St. Louis, MO: C. V. Mosby.

Piggot, L.R. (1979). Overview of selected basic research in autism. *J Autism Dev Disord*, *9*, 199-218.

Ramm, P. A. (1983). The occupational therapy process in specific pediatric conditions. In H.L. Hopkins & H.D. Smith (Eds.), *Willard and Spackman's occupational therapy* (6th ed., pp. 589-641). Philadelphia PA: J.B. Lippincott.

Reilly, C., Nelson, D., & Bundy, A. (1983). Sensorimotor versus fine motor activities in eliciting vocalizations in autistic children. *Occup Ther J of Research*, *3*(4), 199-212.

Rimland, B. (1964). *Infantile autism*. New York: Century Crofts.

Rutter, M. (1978). Diagnosis and definition of childhood schizophrenia. *J Autism Child Schizophr*, *8*, 139-161.

Schanzenbacher, K.E. (1985). Diagnostic problems in pediatrics. In P. Clark & A. S. Allen (Eds.), *Occupational therapy for children* (pp. 78-110). St. Louis, MO: C.V. Mosby.

Schlopler, E. (1965). Early infantile autism and receptor processes. *Arch Gen Psychiatry*, *113*, 1183-1189.

Student, M., & Sohmer, H. (1978). Evidence from auditory nerve and brainstem evoked responses for an organic brain lesion in children with autistic traits. *J Autism Child Schizophr*, *8*, 13-20.

Tiffany, E. (1983). Psychiatry and mental health. In H.L. Hopkins & H.D. Smith (Eds.), *Willard and Spackman's occupational therapy* (6th ed.) (pp. 267-333). Philadelphia, PA: J. B. Lippincott.

Weston, D. (1960). Therapeutic Crafts. *Am J Occup Ther*, *14*, 121-122.

Weston, C. (1961). The dimensions of crafts. *Am J Occup Ther, 15,* 1-5.
Weyman, P., & Abramson, M. (1976). Three theoretical approaches to play: Applications for exceptional children. *Am J Occup Ther, 30,* 551-558.
Wing, L. (1976). *Early childhood autism.* New York: Pergamon Press.
Wolkowicz, R., Fish, J., & Schaffer, R. (1977). Sensory integration with autistic children. *Can J Occup Ther, 44*(4), 171-175.

Going to the Source:
The Use of Qualitative Methodology in a Study of the Needs of Adults with Cerebral Palsy

Alice Kibele, MS, OTR
Lela A. Llorens, PhD, OTR/L, FAOTA

SUMMARY. A small but growing body of occupational therapy literature identifies the value of qualitative research methodology, which is useful with relatively unstudied or complex phenomena. This paper describes the use of qualitative research to obtain insight into the world of adults with significantly limiting cerebral palsy, as seen from their own perspective. The first author conducted extended, guided interviews with five adults who live independently with attendant care. The resulting data, synthesized into recurring themes, suggested guidelines for occupational therapy practice. In this paper, the study methodology is described in depth, and directions for further qualitative and quantitative research are presented.

A growing number of authors have cited the value of qualitative research as a valid source of information to direct occupational therapy practice (Yerxa, 1983; Kielhofner, 1982, 1983; Merrill, 1985). Merrill (1985) clarified that while quantitative methods facilitate

Alice Kibele is Director of Occupational Therapy, Children's Hospital at Stanford, 520 Sand Hill Road, Palo Alto, CA 94304. Lela A. Llorens is Professor, Chair and Graduate Coordinator, Department of Occupational Therapy, San Jose State University, One Washington Square, San Jose, CA 95192-0059.

The authors acknowledge the assistance of Karen Diasio Serrett, Gordon Burton, and Edward V. Roberts in the preparation of the study.

The study on which this paper is based was completed in partial fulfillment of the requirements for the degree, Master of Sciences, completed by the first author at San Jose State University, May, 1986.

analysis of known relationships, qualitative methods allow discovery of previously unknown relationships. Quantitative measures are used to compare the outcomes of treatment approaches and the utilization of particular devices or adaptations, when those approaches, devices and adaptations are known to the researcher. Quantitative methodology is used to test existing theories.

Qualitative methodology is used when the phenomena to be studied represent a larger, unknown entity, such as a culture. Adults with significantly limiting physical disability such as cerebral palsy who live independently with attendant care represent a culture about which there is little documented research. The purpose of this paper is to present the qualitative methodology used in a study that sought to define the needs of adults with significantly limiting cerebral palsy.

There is a small body of occupational therapy literature which defines aspects of intervention with infants and children who have cerebral palsy. Adults with significantly limiting cerebral palsy represent a population about which little is known, and little has been written in occupational therapy or other literature to describe their needs.

DESCRIPTION OF THE STUDY

Study Rationale

The study described here was undertaken to obtain insight into the world of adults with significantly limiting cerebral palsy, who have had experience with services provided in traditional medical/rehabilitation settings and in independent living skills agencies.

Interest in this population was heightened by the first author's clinical experience as an occupational therapy consultant to community-based, publicly-funded agencies serving individuals with developmental disabilities and their families. The first author was introduced to numbers of adults with significantly limiting cerebral palsy who had successfully made a transition from living situations in which all their care needs were met, to the less restrictive environment of independent living with attendant care. Other adults, with similar or milder symptoms of cerebral palsy, continued to live in restrictive environments, while expressing a desire to be more independent. An overriding question for the first author was the role that experiences with services, including occupational therapy, had played in the lives of those who had successfully made that transition.

It was also clear that knowledge about the special culture of childhood and adulthood of people with cerebral palsy is needed by occupational therapists and others who serve this population. In Kielhofner (1983), Yerxa noted that an understanding of the patient's sources of satisfaction and view of himself in his world is critical to insuring active participation of the patient in therapeutic goal-setting and decision-making.

A number of authors, including Kielhofner (1983), cited the importance of competency behaviors in the developmental progression from childhood to independent, satisfying adulthood. The first author of the current study was fascinated to know more about the development of adults with severe motor disabilities, for whom competency as we know it in many basic developmental skills had never occurred. In Kielhofner (1983), Kielhofner and Miyake proposed a "relativity theory of competence." They suggest that in order to define a good performance for an individual with function radically altered by disease or disability, one must acknowledge "the perspective (however limited or deviant) of the individual and the ability of another to recognize and appreciate performance from the same perspective" (page 262).

The first author's observations from outside the world of the study population and a review of literature generated insufficient information on which to base hypotheses that could be studied quantitatively. A number of questions were raised, however, that were appropriate for qualitative study. The following were among the identified questions:

1. What is the role of occupational therapy with adults who are significantly limited by cerebral palsy?
2. What are the perceptions of adults with significantly limiting cerebral palsy regarding their needs for assistance to achieve and maintain independent living?

Selection of Subjects

The participants who contributed data for the study are five adults, three males and two females, who live independently with attendant care in densely populated, urban and suburban neighborhoods of Alameda County, in the San Francisco Bay area of California. They ranged in age from thirty-five to forty-seven at the time the interviews were conducted. The two female participants are married to men with similar physical disabilities; of the males, one counts a similarly-disabled male roommate as his significant other. One male lives with an able-bodied female friend and an able-bodied male attendant. The final subject, a male, lives with an able-bodied, female attendant.

All participants have been diagnosed as having cerebral palsy by the physicians they identified as most knowledgeable about their care. All are caucasian. Three participants rely solely on public financial assistance, which consists of social security, supplemental social security (SSI), and MediCal (California's version of Medicaid). The county pays for a limited number of hours of attendant care for three of the participants. One participant, employed full-time, and another whose husband is a full-time employee, are ineligible for any public financial assistance.

All participants are significantly limited in at least two of the following areas: mobility, communication, and use of the hands for functional tasks, including self-care. All rely on attendant care to maintain their independence in the community.

None of the participants displayed evidence of other significantly limiting disability. They varied in terms of cognitive potential or intellect, as evidenced by verbal expression and ability to conceptualize. However, all were able to relate meaningful experience relative to the interview questions, and all evidenced sufficient intellect and functional ability to manage independent community living with attendant care. The first author had had contact prior to initiation of the study with three of the participants. Contact with two had been made on a professional basis at the time of their moves from a sheltered living situation to independent living with attendant care. The first author had been closely involved in those moves, addressing issues including identification of community resources, durable medical equipment and training of new attendants. In addition, the first author had been previously invited to share in birthday celebrations and other social occasions in the homes of those participants. The third study participant previously known to the first author was a co-worker in a publicly-funded agency providing case management services and funding for individuals with developmental disabilities.

Names of the two remaining study participants were obtained following consultation with a community agency involved in consumer-initiated research addressing the needs of individuals with a variety of disabilities. Those two participants were previously unknown.

Prior knowledge of and social ease with study participants is consistent with qualitative, ethnographic research, in which the researcher seeks to become emersed in the daily lives and culture of members of the population being studied (Kielhofner, 1981; Sharrott in Kielhofner, 1983).

DEVELOPMENT OF THE INTERVIEW GUIDELINE

The first author developed the interview guideline based on clinical experience and review of the literature (see Appendix). The general areas to be queried were determined according to their appropriateness or relevance to the ability of individuals with disabilities to live independently. Those general headings finally selected included: living situation (present and past); systems and service delivery (independent living and medical/rehabilitation services, including occupational therapy); childhood; family; relationships with others; life tasks (including self-care, work/volunteer experience, and use of leisure time); and self-description.

Under each general heading was a list of specific questions, designed to guide the recollections of the study participant. Final revisions to the instrument followed review by occupational therapy peers, the thesis advisor, and readers, including an individual significantly limited by a disability other than cerebral palsy.

DATA COLLECTION

Following initial introduction of the study goals and general outline of the interview, each individual was asked to sign an agreement to be a study participant. The participant was also asked to sign a consent form which allowed the first author to seek confirmation of diagnosis from the participant's physician.

Data were gathered by means of extended non-directed interviews, conducted by the first author, using the interview outline described above. Each interview session lasted from one and one half to three and one half hours. Sessions were scheduled in locations such as the participants' homes and place of employment. Sessions were scheduled at the mutual convenience of the first author and participants, and occurred in sequence until all interview questions had been addressed.

As is typical of phenomenological methodology, the intent of the study was to create a broadly-based outline to guide the interview process. During the actual interview process, conversation with study participants frequently strayed from the outline, as they offered insights on matters of particular importance to them. In such instances, the interview outline served as a framework to which the interviewer and participant returned. The interview insured a legitimate data base, since all participants were given the opportunity to respond to the same questions.

In addition, the interview sessions changed with each succeeding session, in instances when participants offered unsolicited information of obvious value to them. When such new information was offered, the first author restructured subsequent interview sessions to allow sharing of experience regarding the same subject by the other participants.

For example, the first author did not initially include interview questions specifically about sexuality. However, when discussing relationships, self-care tasks, and unmet needs, a number of participants volunteered valuable insights regarding their own sexuality. Because interviews with the five participants were conducted concurrently, but were initiated sequentially, the first author was able to incorporate additional questions for subsequent sessions with other participants to encourage sharing of their insights about sexuality.

With participants' prior knowledge and consent, interviews were audio recorded and the participants' responses were repeated in order to assure that the responses were adequately recorded, and to ease later transcription of data.

There were a total of forty-two interview sessions for all five participants, ranging from six sessions for one participant to eleven sessions for another. The average number of interview sessions per participant was 8.4, with an average of 15.7 total hours spent in interviews with each participant. Total time spent in interviews was just over 80 hours.

Interview sessions were informal, and often included the sharing of a snack or coffee with the participant, as well as informal discussion with the participant and others present (spouses, attendants, friends), either prior to or at the conclusion of the interview sessions. Such informal socialization, and accompanying two of the participants to local restaurants for meals following a number of interview sessions gave additional insight into relevant issues, including the participants' interactions with strangers, and the everyday challenges of environmental accessibility. This collection of data pertaining to a single issue from several sources is referred to as triangulation (Kielhofner, 1982; Merrill, 1985), and strengthens the study's validity.

DATA ANALYSIS

Audio recorded interviews were transcribed verbatim by the first author, with interview questions lending form and order to the content. With the transcription process completed, typewritten copies of each participant's responses were cut into sections, to allow compilation of data from all participants in response to interview guideline sections and specific questions.

The text of the data section was then prepared by noting participants' responses to each section and question in turn. Relevant information was also included that was noted following informal interviews with participants' significant others and attendants, and during outings with participants. During the course of preparation of the text, and across the boundaries of specific areas of the interviews with all participants, the first author noted recurrence of similar ideas, often stated by participants with particular fervor. Notes were made of each such important observation or statement on an individual note care. At the time of completion of the data compilation into typewritten form, there existed a sizeable collection of cards, each bearing a particularly interesting observation.

Those individual observations were next grouped for similarity, using the "storyboard" format advanced by Kemp (1977), to allow easy visualization of all individual notecards in an organized fashion, and at the same time. From organization of these observations there emerged the following eight recurring themes: the universality of experience, similarity to other minorities, the significance of purposeful activity, the hierarchy of disability, the disability as the enemy, dependency versus independence, the importance of control of one's life, and the importance of the attitude of others. The recurring themes provided the major source for information to answer the original study questions, and suggested implications for occupational therapy practice and research.

DISCUSSION OF DATA

This discussion focuses on a brief description of limited sections of the data generated by the methodology; a detailed discussion of the results regarding occupational therapy services are presented elsewhere (see Kibele, accepted for publication, AJOT, 1988). Although the original intent of the research was to describe a role for occupational therapists who work with adults with cerebral palsy, important implications emerged as well for practice with children.

Generally, all participants remembered having received therapy services (occupational, physical, and speech therapy). Early experiences with device-assisted mobility were among their best memories of therapy services. Worst memories included isolation from non-disabled peers, therapists who presented "professional," non-caring or judgmental attitudes, pain, fear of falling, and a perception of personal failure when goals of therapy remained unmet.

They recalled the personalities and intervention styles of specific therapists, and recalled as helpful those who had regarded them as people who happened to have a disability. In addition, therapists were regarded as helpful who had engaged the participants and their families in the decision-making process.

According to the participants, occupational therapists who serve them in medical/rehabilitation and independent living services agencies provide a valuable service when they help individuals with cerebral palsy identify and capitalize on inner resources, acknowledge constraints to the achievement of independence, and overcome or compensate for environmental and societal barriers to independent living.

A number of opportunities for further occupational therapy qualitative and quantitative research emerged from the study. Replication of this study is appropriate, either in the same geographical area, or in an area where both medical/rehabilitation and independent living services differ from those offered in the area where the study was conducted.

Further review of gathered data combined with data from similar studies may yield information about the impact of significantly limiting physical disability on adaptation. Such research can yield additional information about the value of work and leisure experience for individuals born with disabilities. Research remains to be conducted regarding the relationship between attendants and the disabled adults they serve. Issues related to utilization of and relationship with adaptive equipment need further exploration. Specific topics include the relationship between the individual and his or her wheelchair, the physiological and psychological consequences of restraint, and the relationship between wheelchair positioning and function.

Another area for research involves the impact on the developing child and adolescent of constant handling for therapy and attention to care needs. What is the impact of that handling on the child's or adult's ability to learn to play, establish relationships and distinguish loving or sexual touch from other forms of touch? Although the issue has been addressed by some authors, including Vash (1981), occupational therapy can contribute information of value for theory and practice.

In a similar fashion, research is needed to understand and appreciate the perceived physical and psychological pain the study participants recalled in association with therapy they had received as children. Further study is needed to assure that such fear, discomfort, and perceived loss of control are minimized.

Responses of several participants revealed the need for further contribution by occupational therapy to research related to sexuality. Occupational therapists have knowledge of positioning, functional adaptation, and psychological issues involved in sexuality which are needed by individuals with such physical limitations.

Research remains to be conducted regarding differences between persons born with disabilities and those whose disabilities are acquired later in life. Knowledge of such differences, where they exist relative to life satisfaction and adaptation will be useful to clinical practitioners, and has the potential to increase the effectiveness of therapy intervention.

Occupational therapy research will serve a vital purpose if it is able to determine the association among such variables as increased independence, readiness for employment, and costs of care among persons with limiting physical disabilities. The needs of such individuals for attendant services and environmental adaptations do not always represent substantial savings over institutional care. However, therapists are in a position to conduct research that offers convincing evidence about quality of life issues.

Finally, data gathered in this study can serve as a standard against which to measure successful adaptation of future adults now exposed to the occupational therapy intervention of the 1980s.

CONCLUSION

This paper has presented the qualitative methodology used in a study which sought feedback about their needs from five adults with significantly limiting cerebral palsy who live independently with attendant care. Results of the study add to the small but growing body of qualitative research by occupational therapists that attempts to understand the world of individuals with disabilities from their own, unique perspective. An understanding of that perspective provides a vital component of a frame of reference for the provision of occupational therapy services, and directs future, relevant occupational therapy research.

REFERENCES

Kemp, J. (1977). *Instructional Design: A Plan for Unit and Course Development.* Belmont, CA: Fearon-Pitman.

Kielhofner, G. (1981). An ethnographic study of deinstitutionalized adults: Their community settings and daily life experiences. *Occupational Therapy Journal of Research, 1,* 125-146.

Kielhofner, G. (1982). Qualitative research: Part one. The paradigmatic grounds and issues of reliability and validity. *Occupational Therapy Journal of Research. 2,* 67-79.

Kielhofner, G. (1983). *Health through occupation: Theory and practice in occupational therapy.* Philadelphia: F. A. Davis.

Kielhofner, G. & Miyake, S. (1983). Rose-colored lenses for clinical practice: From a deficit to a competency model in assessment and intervention. In Kielhofner, G. (Ed.), *Health through occupation: Theory and practice in occupational therapy* (pp. 257-266). Philadelphia: F. A. Davis.

Merrill, S. (1985). Qualitative methods in occupational therapy research: An application. *Occupational Therapy Journal of Research. 5,* 209-222.

Sharrott, G. (1983). Occupational therapy's role in the client's creation and affirmation of meaning. In Kielhofner, G. (Ed.), *Health through occupation: Theory and practice in occupational therapy* (pp. 213-235). Philadelphia: F. A. Davis.

Vash, C. (1981). *The psychology of disability.* New York: Springer.

Yerxa, E. (1983). Audacious values: The energy source for occupational therapy practice. In G. Keilhofner (Ed.), *Health through occupation: Theory and practice in Occupational therapy* (pp. 149-162). Philadelphia: F. A. Davis.

APPENDIX
INTERVIEW GUIDELINES

Living Situation

Have you ever lived in a large residential facility? If so, what was that like?

Tell me a little bit about the places you have lived.

Describe the situation where you now live. What is good about it? What would you like to change?

Describe the ideal living situation for you. What would you like to have in your environment?

What resources are available to you to help get you into your ideal living situation? What gets in the way of that? If your living situation is ideal, what persons or systems were beneficial in helping you get there?

Systems and Service Delivery

Describe your education. To what extent do you feel it has prepared you for your life as an adult?

As a child and adolescent, did you receive physical, occupational and/ or speech therapy? Where received (location and system), and for how long?

Have you received any therapy services as an adult? When, where and describe.

What was therapy like? What do you remember as the best thing about therapy? The worst?

As an adult, how is the medical care you receive? Are you satisfied that your doctor knows your needs?

If you have been hospitalized as a child, or as an adult, what was that experience like?

Have you had orthopedic surgery? Other surgery? Your view of the value of that surgery?

What do you need most in terms of medical care? What is most helpful to you in getting that care? What (if anything) seems to get in the way of obtaining that care?

Have you had contact with any Independent Living Skills assistance agency? If so, tell me about the services provided, and the appropriateness/helpfulness of those services? How did you gain access to those services?

Are your financial resources adequate? The source of your money?

Childhood

Describe your earliest memories.

Did you spend time with other children when you were small? Were they disabled or able-bodied?

What did you choose to do with free time when you were a child? As an adolescent?

Describe your adolescence.

Family

What was your family like? How was it growing up with them? Did your disability effect them? If so, in what ways?

How did your parents treat you when you were a child? An adolescent?

What were your responsibilities as a child? Your privileges? Did those change with adolescence?

If your parents are still alive and you have contact with them, what is the nature of your relationship now?

Do you have brothers and sisters? How do you think they were affected by your disability? What was your relationship like with them when you were a child; an adolescent; and now, as an adult?

How was it to be a person with a disability in an able-bodied family?

Relationships with Others

What relationships do you currently have with other disabled persons? With able-bodied persons?

Do you associate more with other disabled persons, or with the able-bodied? Is that by choice or circumstance?

Describe your most memorable, or most important relationship (current or past).

How do strangers treat you? Are your experiences generally positive or negative?

Are there circumstances under which you are unaware, or only minimally aware of your disability? more aware?

Describe the differences (if they exist) between your relationships with strangers and with those to whom you are no longer unfamiliar.

Life Tasks

Describe a typical, 24-hour day for you.

Tell me about the things you are currently able to do for yourself, and the things others must help you with, or do for you. Can you rate those tasks according to their significance to you? What is it like to need help with personal (and not so personal) tasks?

What adaptive equipment do you need? Do you have? Tell me a little about the process of getting it. Who/what was helpful? In what ways were or are you hindered from getting the adaptive equipment you need?

Is your personal care adequate for you? If not, what limits the care you receive? Does it relate to skills you don't have but could learn? Does it relate to financial assistance, or to attendants who work for you? Anything else?

Give me a rough estimate of the amount of personal care time you require (including things you do for yourself, and things others do for you).

Are you currently employed (paid for work)? Do you do volunteer work (unpaid)? If so, describe what you do. How much of your time is devoted to work or volunteering?

If you are employed or volunteer your time, describe the process of finding/qualifying for work. What is your employment history?

What is the meaning for you of your work?

If you are not employed or volunteering time, would you like to be? What is the significance of work for you?

What is your favorite way to spend your spare (or leisure) time? Actual experience? Fantasy?

What ways (other than your favorite) do you spend your leisure time?

How much of your time would you say is devoted to leisure? Is that comfortable for you?

What would you characterize as your greatest unmet needs? What is preventing you from attaining satisfaction of those needs?

What are the things/people/events in your life right now, with which you are most satisfied.

Self-Description

Describe yourself to me; or, how do you view yourself?

Do you view yourself as disabled? or, describe your disability.

Have you ever thought about, or reflected on, why you are disabled? Please share that thinking with me.

In what ways are you most disabled?

Are there any ways in which your disability works for you? Do you, or have you ever, used your disability to get what you want?

What are your greatest strengths? or, what are the best things you have going for you?

REPEAT GOALS OF STUDY and ask if there is anything else subject would like to add that would aid researcher's understanding of the topic.

Occupational Therapy and Epilepsy

Carol Maier Clerico, OTR

SUMMARY. Epilepsy and its varied seizure types effect the physical, social, emotional, recreational and vocational functioning of individuals and their families. This article addresses the various components of seizure disorders and discusses the importance of occupational therapy intervention in each of these areas. Epilepsy first aid, safety and activities of daily living, and the role of the occupational therapist in education and vocational exploration are discussed, along with a concise description of epilepsy and its seizure types.

INTRODUCTION

Occupational therapy with individuals who have seizure disorders is both one of the most challenging and one of the most rewarding practice areas today. Unlike any other treatment area, epilepsy presents the therapist with the opportunity to use nearly all of the broad range of occupational therapy knowledge and skills.

Although seizures come in many forms and are frequently associated with other disorders, the very nature of epilepsy implies the potential for deficits in physical, emotional, social, vocational and recreational arenas. The therapist must have an understanding of seizure types, complications, clinical manifestations and behavioral

Carol Maier Clerico is Director of Rehabilitation Services, Martha Jefferson Hospital, 459 Locust Avenue, Charlottesville, VA 22901. Prior to assuming this position, Ms. Clerico was Director of Occupational/Physical/Recreational Therapy at Blue Ridge Hospital, University of Virginia where she worked with the Comprehensive Epilepsy Center for seven years.

The author wishes to thank Nancy Santilli, Ruth Goldeen, and Denise Dulaney of the University of Virginia Comprehensive Epilepsy Center and Bonnie Kessler of the Epilepsy Foundation of America for their assistance.

responses before effective treatment techniques can be selected. Consequently, this article will include a short description of epilepsy and seizure types before discussing the role of the occupational therapist with this complicated disorder.

DESCRIPTION OF EPILEPSY AND SEIZURE TYPES

An individual is considered to have epilepsy when he or she has had two or more seizures not precipitated by fever, infection, metabolic disease or toxin (Black, Hermann, and Shope, 1982). The Epilepsy Foundation of America estimates that one in every 100 adults and one in every 50 school age children has epilepsy (personal communication, 1988). The causes of epileptic seizures are many and varied. Stimulation of a group of cells in the brain can cause these cells to develop a sudden burst of hyperactivity. If this activity reaches a high enough magnitude, it may spread throughout the nervous system causing seizures (Sands, 1982).

The classification of epilepsy has two major components: (1) partial seizures, which begin in a specific part of the brain and usually start with symptoms limited to a local part of the body or a single function, and (2) generalized seizures, which begin in the whole brain. The international classification of seizure types and the corresponding EEG activity may be seen in Figures 1 and 2, adapted from Santilli (1987).

The following descriptions of the most common seizure types are adapted from Holmes (1987), Dreifuss(1983), Sands (1982), and Black, Hermann, and Shope (1982).

Partial Seizures

Partial seizures are subdivided into elementary (simple) types, which do not involve impaired consciousness, and complex types, in which consciousness is impaired. Partial seizures may spread to become generalized seizures, but their focal beginning is important for proper diagnosis and appropriate therapy.

The complications, clinical manifestations, and behavioral responses of partial seizures depend upon the part of the brain affected by the injury or insult. The therapist will observe a wide range of responses that vary with seizure type.

Simple Partial Seizures with Motor Signs

These seizures are the most common type of simple partial seizures. Characterized by tonic or clonic movements of muscles, these seizures will affect any body part depending on the site of origin on the motor strip. The seizure may involve only small muscle groups, such as twitching of a finger or small muscles of the mouth, or may involve larger muscle groups, such as seen with clonic movements of an entire extremity. These clonic movements may progress to involve the whole of one side of the body. Occasionally, the seizure may be associated with decreased tone and the extremity may be flaccid.

Focal seizures are commonly characterized by adversive movements, such as turning the head or eyes toward one side of the body. A simple partial seizure with a progressive march of sensations or movements from one body part to another is called a Jacksonian seizure.

Following partial motor seizures, temporary paralysis of the muscle groups involved in the seizure, called Todd's paralysis, may last from several minutes up to several hours. Aphasia may also occur under several conditions with partial seizures. A partial seizure may remain focal or may progress to impaired consciousness and become a complex partial seizure.

Simple Partial Seizures with Autonomic Sensations

Pupil dilatation is probably the most common autonomic sensation in simple seizures. Other seizures include "goose bumps," stomachache, vomiting, pallor or flushing, sweating, palpitations, or salivation.

Simple Partial Seizures with Sensory Symptoms

Seizures arising from the parietal lobe often begin with vague to specific sensations, including paresthesias, numbness, and somatosensory symptoms. Rarely are these sensations painful, usually being reported as merely disturbing and sometimes unpleasant. Some individuals report a sensation of distortion of body parts, such as a

FIGURE 1. Classification of Epileptic Seizures, Partial — Adapted from Santilli (1987)

Seizure Type	EEG Type
A. Simple Partial – Consciousness not impaired	Local contralateral discharges starting over the corresponding area of cortical representation

1. Motor
  a. focal motor without march
  b. focal motor with march (Jacksonian)
  c. versive
  d. postural
  e. phonatory (arrest of speech or vocalization)
2. Autonomic (pallor, epigastric sensation sweating, piloerection flushing, and pupillary dilation)
3. Somatosensory (simple hallucinations)

Seizure Type	EEG Type

unreality)
  d. affective (fear, anger, and other emotional states)
  e. illusions (macropsia)
  f. structural hallucinations (hear a specific song or see a detailed scene)

B. Complex Partial – With alteration of consciousness	Unilateral or bilateral diffuse or focal discharge in temporal or fronto-temporal regions

1. Simple partial→Complex partial
  a. simple partial features followed by impairment of consciousness
  b. simple partial

a. visual (flashing lights)
b. auditory (buzzing)
c. somatosensory (tingling)
d. olfactory (unpleasant odor)
e. gustatory (pleasant or odious taste)
f. vertiginous (falling in space, floating)
4. Psychic symptoms
a. dysphasia
b. dysmnesia (deja vu, distorted memory, forced thinking)
c. cognitive (dreamy state, detachment,

features followed by automastism
2. Impairment of consciousness at onset
a. only seizure feature
b. automatisms
3. Partial seizures that secondarily generalize
a. simple partial→ generalized tonic-clonic
b. complex partial→ generalized tonic-clonic
c. simple partial→ complex partial→ generalized tonic-clonic

Discharge like those for partial seizures that then rapidly generalize

Adapted from Commission on Classification and Terminology of the International League Against Epilepsy.

FIGURE 2. Classification of Epileptic Seizures, Generalized — Adapted from Santilli (1987)

Seizure Type	EEG Type
A. Absence (petit mal) 1. Typical absence a. impairment of consciousness b. mild clonic components c. atonic components d. tonic components e. autonomic components	Regular and symmetrical, bilateral abnormalities, usually 3 Hz activity, but may be 2–4 Hz spike and wave complexes, background activity usually normal
2. Atypical absence a. pronounced body tone changes b. onset/cessation not abrupt	Irregular and asymmetrical, bilateral abnormalities, more heterogenous, irregular spike and slow wave complexes, fast activity, background activity usually abnormal
B. Tonic-clonic (grand mal)	10 or more cycles per second, tonic phase-decreased frequency and increased amplitude, clinic phase-slow waves
C. Myoclonic (single or multiple, short, abrupt muscle contractions)	Polyspike and wave discharges spike and wave, sharp and slow wave
D. Clonic (muscle contraction and relaxation)	At least 10 cycles per second (fast activity) and slow waves
E. Tonic (muscle contraction)	Low voltage, fast activity or fast rhythm (9–10 cycles per second), decreasing in frequency and increasing in amplitude
F. Atonic (abrupt loss of muscle tone)	Polyspikes and wave discharges flattening, low-voltage fast activity

Adapted from Commission on Classification and Terminology of the International League Against Epilepsy.

feeling of changing extremity size or a sense of absence of a body part. Occasionally, atonicity may occur in a portion of the extremity. Usually, focal cortical seizures last for only a few seconds or a few minutes.

Simple partial seizures with special sensory phenomena may include olfactory symptoms such as distortions of smell, usually unpleasant odors. These olfactory symptoms may be the only seizure manifestation, or may be followed by motor activity and an altered state of consciousness, leading to a complex partial seizure.

Gustatory sensations with simple partial seizures vary from tastes that are described as pleasant to "metallic." Auditory seizures vary greatly from simple sounds such as rushing and hissing to complex phenomenon such as recognizable music or sounds of familiar events. Vertiginous seizures include sensations of falling and floating, as well as dizziness. Visual seizures arising from the occipital lobe vary greatly in magnitude and description. Flashing lights, hallucinations of people and places, sensations of darkness or unstructured spectral visualizations, shapes, animals, or panoramic hallucinations may occur. Occipital lobe seizures frequently progress to complex partial seizures or tonic-clonic seizures.

The partial seizure is often called an aura, as it may be a warning of impending complex partial seizures or generalized tonic-clonic seizures, and is often the only part of the seizure recalled by the individual.

Simple Partial Seizures with Dysmnesic Symptoms or Cognitive Disturbances

Distortion of time sense, a dreamy state, or the sensations of deja vu or jamais vu may represent another type of simple seizure. Cognitive disturbances, including sensations of unreality, detachment, or depersonalization may also be present. Sensations of pleasure or displeasure, fear, depression, unprovoked anger that abates quickly, illusions, or structured hallucinations may also occur with simple partial seizures.

Complex Partial Seizures

"The cardinal point that separates complex partial seizures from simple partial seizures is the impairment, distortion, or loss of the conscious state'' (Dreifuss, 1983). Complex partial seizures are one of the most common seizure types that occur in children. Since the focus of most complex partial seizures is the temporal lobe, an area concerned with memory and emotion, clinical symptoms may be quite complex and variable, encompassing the entire range of neuropsychiatric symptoms (Pedley and Meldrum, 1985). Because of the frequency of focus in the temporal lobe, and the automatic behaviors often exhibited during complex partial seizures, they have previously been called temporal lobe or psychomotor seizures.

Some individuals are aware of impending seizures hours or even days before the event. Seizure prodrome may consist of headaches, insomnia, irritability, unexplained feelings of fear or depression, or changes in personality or activity level.

As discussed earlier, a simple partial seizure may precede the loss of consciousness of the complex partial seizure. This ''aura'' is the part of the seizure experienced before consciousness is lost and is often the only part of the seizure individuals remember following recovery from the full seizure. Auras may include visual, auditory, labyrinthine, or cognitive signs. These include misperceptions of size and distance, changing sounds, disturbances in spacial awareness, or feelings of changing time sense or unreality. Hallucinatory phenomena may occur. Somatosensory symptoms, as well as subjective experiences, have also been reported.

Automatisms (unconscious, automatic behaviors, frequently occurring with complex partial seizures) occur when consciousness is impaired either during the ictal or postictal period. The individual is either amnesic or partially amnesic for these phenomena. Automatisms may be perseverative in nature, continuing activities in progress prior to the seizure, or may be new activities, responding to some stimuli, or may be activities that are usually atypical for the individual.

Automatisms may be alimentary, including chewing, lip or tongue smacking, or swallowing. Mimicry automatisms are facial expressions that reflect fear, anxiety, anger, or joy and may be accompanied by utterances. Gestural automatisms include clapping, scratching, and other repetitive hand movements. They may include quasipurposeful movements, such as playing music, cleaning, polishing, or drawing. Automatisms of an ambulatory nature may include walking, running, or riding a bicycle (and avoiding objects), and may be goal-directed or disorganized. Verbal automatisms include screaming, crying, laughing, or repeating phrases. Some autonomic symptoms such as abdominal pain may be associated with complex partial seizures (Dreifuss, 1983; Holmes, 1987).

People with complex partial seizures frequently complain of problems with memory. Sometimes a loss of memory precedes a loss of consciousness, and may serve as an aura for the individual having the seizure.

Affective symptoms may include feelings of fear and sadness, depression, embarrassment, or joy and excitation. Rage attacks have been reported and may be associated with hyperkinetic syndrome in children. Gelastic, or laughing seizures, elicit a laugh different from spontaneous, natural laughter, and individuals with gelastic seizures express feelings of fear or dread prior to the seizure, rather than mirth. Speech abnormalities, including speech arrest and expressive aphasia are common in complex partial seizures. Cognitive disturbances, illusions, and hallucinations have also been reported.

Complex partial seizures may also arise in the frontal lobe. These seizures are difficult to distinguish from temporal lobe seizures, but lack the affective signs and psychic symptoms, and have increased frequency of motor phenomena. Motor activity may include deviations of head and eyes, falls, or increased or decreased muscle tone (Holmes, 1987).

Generalized Seizures

Generalized seizures are those without local onset, and reflect a larger hyperexcitability or instability of the brain. (Sands, 1982) They include absence, myoclonis, infantile spasms, tonic, clonic, or tonic-clonic, atonic, and akinetic seizures. Generalized seizures result in a marked impairment of consciousness.

Absence Seizures

Absence seizures are characterized by rhythmic, generalized, three per second spike and wave discharge. The seizures are short, lasting approximately 15-30 seconds involving a brief loss of consciousness and may include staring, eye fluttering, and twitching of mouth or hands. Absence seizures, as classified by Dreifuss (1983), include absence seizures with impairment of consciousness alone, with mild clonic components, with atonic components, with tonic components, with automatisms, and with autonomic components. The hallmarks of the absence attack are sudden onset, interruption of ongoing activities, a blank stare, and possibly a brief upward rotation of the eyes (Dreifuss, 1983).

With the simple absence, there is a sudden cessation of activity. The individual becomes transfixed and stares motionless. Normal breathing continues. The eyes become vacant, sometimes with drooping lids, and may then turn upward. There are no other manifestations. Although the individual is unresponsive during the attack, the end of the seizure brings immediate recovery, with a resumption of the activity in progress before the seizure as though nothing had happened. A sentence will be completed or a motion resumed as though there had been no interruption. The individual may be unaware that a seizure has occurred. True simple absence seizures are rare.

Complex absence seizures are much more frequent. Clonic components, including eye blinking, nystagmus, or subtle clonic or myoclonic movements of the arms, hands, or mouth may be evident with complex absence seizures. Absence with changes in postural tone may be evidenced by muscular contractions in a symmetrical or asymmetrical manner causing the individual to lurch forward or arch backward. The head or arms may drop or be pulled to one side. The decreased tone of absence seizures is rarely sufficient to cause the individual to fall. As with complex partial seizures, absence seizures may be accompanied by automatisms or autonomic phenomena.

Myoclonic Seizures

Myoclonic seizures, as described by Dreifuss (1983), are "sudden, brief, shock-like contractions that may be generalized or confined to the face or tongue, or to one or more extremities, or even to individual muscles or groups of muscles." Myoclonic jerks may be rapidly repetitive or relatively isolated. They may occur predominantly around the hours of going to sleep or of awakening from sleep. They may be exacerbated by volitional movements and are then known as action myoclonus. At times, they may be regularly repetitive.

Infantile Spasms

Infantile spasms are to a large degree age specific, occurring during the first two years of life. They are characterized by single or repetitive muscle contractions in flexion or extension. They may be represented by short head nods or full body flexion or extension. They may be accompanied by autonomic manifestations, eye deviation or nystagmus. Spasms may occur singly or in clusters.

Tonic, Clonic, and Tonic-Clonic Seizures

Although they can occur independently, tonic seizures and clonic seizures usually occur in combination in the classic, easily recognized tonic-clonic seizure, previously termed grand mal. Tonic-clonic seizures may be primary and bilaterally symmetrical or they may be secondary to a focal onset. Generalized tonic-clonic seizures may be precipitated by an aura of hours or days.

The tonic-clonic seizure consists of several phases. The seizure begins with a loss of consciousness and a sharp tonic contraction of the muscles. The individual may open the mouth and eyes before falling to the ground in a rigid posture. Respirations are inhibited and cyanosis may occur. A cry may be heard as air is expelled and forced over the vocal cords. The mouth may forcibly close, sometimes causing the individual to bite the tongue. Extension of the back and neck follows. This tonic phase is sometimes called the flexion and extension phase of the seizure (Holmes, 1987). During the brief transition from the tonic to the clonic phase of the seizure, the rigidity may be replaced by a fine tremor. This is sometimes called the tremor phase (Holmes, 1987).

As the tonic phase gives way to the clonic convulsive phase, grunting respirations may be heard between the convulsive movements. During the clonic phase, the muscles intermittently contract and relax, resulting in rhythmic jerks which decrease in frequency as the seizure progresses. The individual may remain cyanotic and saliva may froth from the mouth. At the end of this stage, all muscles relax, including the bladder sphincter, and incontinence may result. The individual usually remains unconscious for varying periods of time. As the individual awakens, confusion and drowsiness may be noted. Some people progress directly into sleep without even waking from the seizure.

The entire sequence noted above will vary in time with the individual lasting from one minute to several minutes.

Atonic Seizures

Atonic (astatic) seizures or drop attacks, sometimes called akinetic petit mal, are very brief (usually a fraction of a second) with loss of muscle tone involving all the postural muscles or only those of the head and neck. The head suddenly falls to the chest, or if postural muscles are affected, the individual slumps to the ground. Although consciousness is lost during the fall, alertness may return by the time the individual hits the floor. Since drop attacks occur without warning and may involve a total loss of muscle tone, the potential for injury from falls is great. The fall usually happens so suddenly that neither the individual nor the observer has time to protect the individual from injury. If seated, the individual may fall forward, injuring the face. Individuals with drop attacks are therefore encouraged to wear a helmet with protective face guards. Drop attacks frequently coincide with myoclonus (called myoclonic-atonic seizures) or with tonic seizures and are observed in children with chronic encephalopathy and mild mental retardation as seen in Lennox-Gastaut syndrome.

Lennox-Gastaut Syndrome

Severe childhood epileptic encephalopathy characterized by a variety of intractable seizure forms including absence and drop attacks, associated with mental retardation, and having an irregular, slow, spike and wave EEG pattern has been described by a large number of seizure combination descriptions. This syndrome is now commonly called Lennox-Gastaut syndrome.

Seizure types are mixed in Lennox-Gastaut with onset between the ages of 1 and 6 years of age. Tonic, tonic-clonic, myoclonic, atypical absence, and atonic seizures are common with this syndrome. A high frequency of seizures, sometimes interspersed with periods of freedom from attack, developmental delays, and mild retardation accompany the seizures in this devastating syndrome. There is a male predominance for the syndrome. Prognosis is poor.

Pseudoseizures

"Pseudoepileptic seizures are paroxysmal episodes of altered behavior" (Holmes, 1987) that resemble true seizures, but lack the clinical, EEG, and physiologic signs of true seizures. Pseudoseizures are most common in female adolescents and children and often occur in combination with true epileptic seizures. A history of personal or familial emotional stress may help with the diagnosis of pseudoseizures. Holmes (1987) states that the experienced observer may be able to differentiate pseudoseizures from epilepsy (see Figure 3).

There are no absolute criteria for diagnosing pseudoseizures. EEG with video may be helpful as will skilled observation of behaviors. Pseudoseizures are frequently seen in children or adults with epileptic seizures where seizure control might threaten personal or familial emotional stability.

MEDICAL/SURGICAL MANAGEMENT
OF SEIZURES

The topic of medical management of epilepsy would comprise an entire textbook by itself. Management spans the fields of neurology, medicine, pharmacology, and surgery. The study of epilepsy is worldwide and has undergone many changes during the past 10 years. New treatment methods, new attitudes and new philosophies have shifted the medical management of epilepsy from seizure control alone to an emphasis on the quality of life. Diagnosis, including seizure history, electroencephalogram (EEG), video monitoring, computerized tomography (CT), positron emission tomography (PET), magnetic resonance imaging (MRI), and prolonged clinical observations now accompany the standard history and physical exam (Santilli and Sierzant, 1987).

FIGURE 3. Criteria Useful for Differentiating Epileptic from Pseudoseizures – Adapted from Homes (1987)

Clinical Data	Pseudo-Seizures	Generalized Tonic Clonic Seizures	Complex Partial Seizures
Changes in seizure frequency with medication change	Rare	Usual	Usual
Increased seizure frequency with stress	Frequently	Occasionally	Occasionally
Combativeness	Common	Rare	Rare
Vulgar language	Frequent	Rare	Rare
Self injury	Rare	Common	Rare
Incontinence	Rare	Common	Unusual
Tongue biting	Rare	Common	Rare
Nocturnal occurrence	Rare	Common	Occasional
Stereotype attacks	Often variable	Little variation	Not identical but usually have similar pattern
Postictal confusion, lethargy, or sleepiness	Rarely	Always	Frequently
EEG: Interictal	Often normal	Frequently abnormal	Frequently abnormal
During attack	Normal	Always abnormal	Usually abnormal

Antiepileptic drugs, used in the smallest amounts possible with the fewest side effects, are the medical management treatment of choice. Antiepileptic drugs control seizures completely for over 50% of persons with epilepsy and reduce seizure frequency for another 20-30%. Twenty percent of those with epilepsy continue to have intractable seizures (Santilli and Sierzant, 1987). Selection of drugs is individualized and based on the seizure type, the side effects of the drug, the half-life of the drug, the cost of the drug, the age of the individual with seizures, and the individual's tolerance and acceptance of the drug.

For the 20% of the U.S. population for whom medical management has not improved disabling seizures, surgery is becoming an increasingly more viable option. Surgery is not recommended for all individuals with seizures, but can be effective for those with clearly delineated, unilateral, anterior temporal lobe foci (Santilli and Sierzant, 1987).

THE ROLE OF THE OCCUPATIONAL THERAPIST

As one would expect, the occupational therapist's role varies with the treatment setting, the seizure type, and the attitudes and behaviors of the individual. Since seizures respect neither age nor place, the therapist may find him/herself working with seizure-prone individuals in the developmental clinic, the school system, the mental health clinic, the acute care hospital, the vocational/rehabilitation center, the corporation, or the community.

The occupational therapist may be involved in the evaluation and diagnostic process when seizures are suspected. The therapist may be part of the interdisciplinary treatment team that assists the patient with seizure control and modification of lifestyle and activity. Evaluation and treatment of school age children with sensorimotor or other neurological deficits from a brain injury or insult is another common role for the occupational therapist. Working with the adolescent in coping with the added social and psychological stresses of seizures, or assisting the adult, whose sudden onset of seizures forces an unanticipated vocational change reflects additional areas for OT intervention. Assisting the corporation to safely modify a work site to enable the hiring or return to work of an employee with seizures, or helping a community become more aware of the nature of epilepsy and less afraid of the effects of seizures are other common areas of involvement for the occupational therapist.

Interviewing the Individual with Epilepsy

Regardless of the area of practice, several common questions must be asked of the individual with epilepsy. The therapist must interview both the individual and the family or caregivers to determine the understanding, acceptance and attitudes of each regarding the seizure disorder. Questions about type and frequency of seizures, the role the individual plays in the family, the individual's and family's satisfaction with the ability of the individual to continue in this role, the effect of the seizures on daily living skills including work and leisure, and in what way the seizures have impacted on the individual's social and emotional well-being must be addressed. Once the therapist understands not only the physical, but the social, psychological, vocational and recreational impact of the disorder on the individual and the family, he or she can begin to determine appropriate occupational therapy intervention strategies.

Evaluation of the Individual with Epilepsy

The initial interview should be followed by a formal evaluation. In addition to the routine OT assessment areas of strength, range, sensation, behaviors, daily living skills, and occupational roles, the therapist must look at several key areas affecting the individual with epilepsy. For the person with a seizure disorder, the major life adjustments appear to be vocational self-sufficiency, social adequacy, and the capacity for independent living (Sands, 1982).

Because problems in school and work are so common, it is important to identify whether deficits in task performance contribute to these problems. Manual skills, hand dominance, attention span, ability to follow instructions, postural balance and bilateral integration, decision-making and problem solving abilities, body scheme and body image, memory, ability to retain information, and motor praxis should be assessed. The ability to structure time and task, to work with others, take direction and evaluate self may also be explored with the individual and family.

Some centers conduct evaluations on an individual, formal one-on-one basis. Others collect the data through individual or group observations during functional and therapeutic activities (Day, 1984). Once the therapist has determined areas of deficit and appropriate areas for treatment, the treatment plan is developed (with the treatment team, the individual, and the family) and therapy begins.

Epilepsy First Aid

One of the biggest concerns for the new therapist working with people with epilepsy is the question "What do I do if he or she has a seizure?" The following first aid principles as described by Santilli (1987), may be helpful.

Nonconvulsive Seizures

Absence (petit mal)

- No first aid measures necessary unless seizures become more involved, i.e., tonic-clonic

Simple partial

- No first aid measures necessary unless seizures become more involved, i.e., complex partial or tonic-clonic

Complex partial (psychomotor)

- Look for medical identification
- Speak calmly and reassuringly to the person
- Remove and guide the individual from hazards
- Stay with the individuals until completely themselves again (confusion follows this seizure)
- Avoid restraining or grabbing the individual unless sudden danger threatens

Convulsive Seizures

Generalized tonic-clonic (grand mal)

- Look for medical identification
- If possible, move the individual into a hazard-free position and remove hazardous objects
- Turn on side to keep airway clear
- Put something soft under the head
- Loosen tight clothing
- Do NOT put anything in mouth
- Call for help if seizure lasts more than 10 minutes or multiple seizures occur together
- After seizure

  - Speak calmly to the person
  - Let individual rest for a short time
  - Do not give anything to eat or drink until fully alert

Activities of Daily Living, Safety and Independence

"The individual with epilepsy can physically appear, and often perform, like anybody else, except during that period of time in which a seizure occurs. The fact that seizures do occur, however, often results in parents or significant others expecting less of the person in relation to home chores, school achievement, involvement in social and recreational activities and so on. In many cases, a person's decision-making capabilities are pre-empted by members of the family" (Sands, 1982). It is at these times that the therapeutic emphasis must focus on the individual's and family's willingness to help the individual become more independent in the decision-making process.

For individuals with seizure disorders, the level of ability to perform functional activities often revolves around safety. Many of the techniques taught by occupational therapists for improving independence in functional activities are applicable to individuals with epilepsy. The most critical component of these tasks is how they may be performed without injury to the individual. Bathing, dressing, hygiene, grooming, and mobility, as well as homemaking, transportation, cooking, and child care must all be approached with an eye toward safety. Although an individual's ability to be independent varies greatly with age and seizure type, many of the safety tips that follow are applicable to a wide range of problems.

It is of critical importance that we encourage infants and children with epilepsy to become independent in daily activities. It is equally important that we encourage adolescents and adults to remain as independent as possible. One of the most difficult tasks to confront the therapist will be to determine the functional level of the individual with seizures and to further assess the extent to which the family or caregivers permit that function in the home.

One of the hardest decisions for caregivers and families of persons with seizures is to decide when to open the safety net wide enough to enable freedom and independence and when to stay close enough to protect the loved one from injury and harm. It is critical for the occupational therapist to help the person and the family evaluate which activities can be performed safely and independently, which activities require assistance and to what degree, and which activities should be avoided.

The therapist must help the family to realize that a child who cannot (or will not) care for his or her own basic needs will be faced with the disapproval of independent peers, the disappointment of family and friends, and will be programmed for life as a dependent adult. The family must realize that although it fears for the child's safety, fostering this dependence will set up a life pattern that precludes independent functioning and deprives the individual of the knowledge that he or she can live a "normal" life despite the inconvenience of seizures.

As with most disabilities, some limitations in performance of daily tasks will result from physical or cognitive deficits that will indeed preclude task independence. Some limitations in daily activities can be modified or eliminated by the use of specific adaptive techniques or equipment. However, some limitations in daily activities are a result of overprotective caregivers, teachers, family and friends whose fear of injury or misunderstanding of epilepsy have led them to "protect" the seizure prone individual from those normal experiences that help develop and maintain independence. This protective attitude not only effects independence in basic self-care, but expands to include many of life's daily living activities.

The following recommendations may be beneficial to help the person with seizures, the family members, the teacher or the therapist to approach daily activities with less fear and apprehension. The first grouping will be helpful for any individual with seizures. The second group addresses specific problems or concerns that are related to age or seizure type.

General Safety Tips

Falls and a brief to lengthy loss of consciousness from seizures that occur during normal activities may result in injuries from hitting objects, losing awareness of location or motion of extremities, or an inability to move away from harm. Because of the potential for injury during seizures of many types, the following safety tips will be applicable to a variety of problems.

Bathing/Toileting:

- Keep water temperatures in the house turned to warm, not hot to avoid burns.
- Always use non-skid strips in the tub or shower.
- Cover all heating units and pad all counter edges.
- Keep all electrical appliances out of the bathroom and away from water.
- Keep the bathroom well ventilated to prevent heat buildup.
- Use only plastic bottles and containers to avoid broken glass.
- When home alone, sponge bathe do not use tub or shower.
- Always check water temperature with hands before stepping into tub or shower.

Dressing:

- Avoid jewelry or accessories with sharp edges.
- Store clothing at an easy to reach height to avoid climbing.

Feeding/Eating:

- Be sure friends and family know how to assist someone who is choking.
- Do not eat while slumping or lying down.
- Avoid foods and drinks that are hot-high temperatures.
- Use a commuter cup with lid and spout for drinking warm liquids.

Recreation:

- Play on soft surfaces such as grass, carpet, or mats whenever possible.
- Stay away from unprotected heat sources or sharp objects.
- Take frequent rest breaks and stay cool.
- Drink plenty of fluids.
- Wear protective eye glasses.
- Use softballs rather than hard balls.
- When swimming, always wear a life jacket or swim with a friend.
- Do exertional activities in a cool room or outdoors at the coolest part of the day.

Homemaking/Home Safety:

- Keep hallways and walkways clear of clutter.
- Secure electrical and telephone wires out of the walkway.
- Pad sharp corners and edges on furniture.
- Use carpeting and padded flooring whenever possible.
- Keep sharps such as knives, scissors, etc. in a special storage place.
- Do not use throw rugs.

Specific Helps for Specific Ages or Seizure Types

Bathing/Toileting:

- For infants and children with seizures, it may be helpful to have two adults to assist with the bath, or you may wish to do a sponge bath outside the tub.

- For infants with mild seizures, a bath sponge that fits under the infant and supports the head above the water level may be helpful.
- For older children who can bathe themselves, stay near the bathroom and keep up a steady conversation with the child and assist only as needed.
- Tub seats, shower seats, or bath benches with safety straps may be helpful to avoid falls into the water.
- For independent adolescents and adults, showers are generally safer, especially when there is a shower seat.
- Periodic checks by a family member or conversation with someone outside the bathroom are good safety precautions even for independent adults.
- Tub safety rails or grab bars are good to assist getting in and out of the tub or shower.

Hygiene/Grooming:

- Do not let children use curling irons or other electrical appliances unattended.
- Have the child use shatter-proof mirrors.
- Hang a mirror at the child's height to avoid the need to climb on stools.
- For adolescents and adults, have someone present when using heated appliances such as curling irons, hair dryers, etc.
- Use only electric razors. Do not use a straight edge.
- Use a vanity mirror to sit while applying makeup, etc.

Dressing:

- Plan ahead assemble clothes and accessories in one area to avoid frequent trips back and forth while dressing.
- Whether you or your child has seizures, dress infants and small children on the floor.
- Avoid using jewelry for infants and young children with seizures.

Feeding/Eating:

- Avoid spills by using non-skid surfaces under plates and cups.

- A scooped dish may help avoid spills if jerking or poor co-ordination is a problem.
- Use a commuter cup to help avoid spills.
- Check an infant's mouth periodically during meals to check for stored food.
- Secure infants and small children in an infant seat or high-chair.
- If seizures include slumping or falling, chairs with armrests are preferred.

Mobility/Travelling:

- Use a stroller to move an infant or child from place to place.
- Always use carseats and seatbelts when travelling.
- Wearing a helmet, if needed, is always recommended.
- Keep all breakables out of easy reach.
- If seizures at night result in falls from bed, put a small mat, pillows, or folded blankets beside the bed to prevent injury.
- Use a bedrail if falls are frequent.
- Alert neighbors as to what to do if they discover the person with seizures wandering outside alone.
- Driving should be avoided unless cleared by the physician and DMV.
- If falls are frequent, padded clothing or knee and elbow pads may be useful.
- A medical alert bracelet or necklace worn at all times is recommended.
- When travelling, carry the name of your medical doctor, your medications, and appropriate phone numbers in your bag.
- If muscle jerks are unexpected, or if loss of muscle tone is frequent, have a "buddy" carry cafeteria trays.

Child Care:

- Take naps when your child takes naps, so you are both rested.
- For infants, use a crib from which the child cannot climb out.

- Change infants on the floor or use a safety strap on a low changing table.
- Do not bathe a child alone if you have seizures.
- Use only warm water for bathing infants and children.
- Use an intercom in the child's room so that you and others may hear him/her.
- Take a child's temperature under the arm.

Recreation:

- It is a good idea to have a buddy present when you engage in exertional activities.
- Avoid tight, overcrowded spaces that are not well ventilated or free of objects.
- Avoid open flames, sit a distance from campfires and stoves.
- It is good to exercise with a buddy who knows epilepsy first aid.

Homemaking/Home Safety:

- Avoid ironing whenever possible. If you must iron, do so when someone else is present. Use an iron with an automatic cut-off.
- Removing burner controls on stoves except during meal preparation may help prevent burns for those with automatisms.
- Keep all non-food items such as cleaning agents out of the kitchen and bathroom, preferably in a locked closet.
- Using plastic and paper cups around the house may decrease breakage.
- Use a microwave with microwave dishes. This avoids the need to handle hot dishes or to reach over or into hot surfaces.
- If you must use a conventional oven, use long oven mitts and wooden oven rack pulls to prevent reaching into the oven.
- At the stove, use the back burners and long pot holders to avoid inadvertently putting your hand on the burner during a seizure.

- Use a dishwasher when possible or wear rubber gloves to wash dishes to decrease the chance for burns.
- Store all items you use at accessible heights. Don't climb.
- Use a cart to transport items including hot foods from one area to another.
- Slide pots and cooking dishes along the countertop to avoid lifting hot liquids or hot pans.
- Use vegetable choppers or food processors for cutting. Use pre-cut canned or frozen foods.
- If falls occur during seizures, use a helmet at all times in the kitchen.
- Use a colander basket inside a pot to cook vegetables, etc. — lift the basket out of the hot water and let the water cool before moving the pot.
- It is best to cook with a buddy in the kitchen. You have help with the preparations and someone to assist you if you have a seizure.

It is a good idea to plan activities ahead and consider areas that might pose a safety problem. Think about how these problems might be avoided or decreased. It is important for the individual with seizures to understand the consequences of attempting activities without an awareness of safety measures. It is important for the parents of children with seizures to teach their youngsters how to assess situations and look for solutions to potential problems. The family must encourage the child to live safely by helping the child to make independent choices and understand the consequences of those choices.

A child must learn to be aware of seizure precautions without always being afraid to try new activities. Parents, teachers, and therapists can foster this attitude by helping the child to understand the immediate consequences of small choices. For example, if a child has drop attacks and falls to the floor during seizures, the parent should not make the child feel that play should be avoided because of possible injury. The parent should talk with the child about the possibility for falling during the drop attacks and the possibility for injury. The parent should then give the child a choice of precautions. Does the child wish to wear a helmet or play on padded surfaces? This choice gives the child a chance to make an independent decision, aware of the consequences, and offers him the chance to engage in normal leisure activity.

The therapist, the family, and the person with seizures must continue to think of safe ways to do the daily activities of home, work, school and leisure. It is important to maintain independence, but accidents and injury are ever threatening problems when seizures are a part of life.

Education and Learning

Epilepsy is a disorder of the brain. It is not surprising then, that the brain dysfunction of epilepsy will be manifested in ways other than seizures. This short paper is insufficient to describe the many manifestations of brain dysfunction in seizure disorders. But the next few paragraphs will describe some of the most frequent symptoms the therapist will observe during the course of treatment.

Learning disabilities, emotional problems, and motor impairments commonly accompanying seizures may be exacerbated by the medications used to assist with seizure control. These complications in the child with epilepsy frequently lead to poor school performance, depression, low self-esteem, and withdrawal. Children with mild seizures, particularly absence seizures, are frequently at a disadvantage in the school environment where subtle disturbances in memory, perceptual disorders, or attention deficits are often not picked up on the standard performance and intelligence tests used in the schools. Additionally, these children may have the same problems as children with other learning disabilities, and they are mistakenly seen as being simply and easily distracted, unable to stay on task, and inattentive. As with other learning disabled children, those with epilepsy learn early in their school careers certain coping skills, including avoidance and absenteeism, that help them avoid recognition. But most coping skills cannot effectively mask the low self-esteem, depression, anxiety and school failure facing many of these children, particularly those with complex seizure problems.

Baseline intelligence may be affected by age of seizure onset, seizure frequency, the etiology of the seizure disorder, and the types of seizures experienced. This impact on baseline intelligence is a critical factor in successful school performance.

Temporal lobe lesions that result in partial complex seizures may directly impair memory functions. Additionally, some antiepileptic medications also affect the memory process. Temporal lobe lesions in the dominant hemisphere may impair verbal abilities and lesions in the non-dominant hemisphere may impair visual-motor or perceptual-motor abilities, as well as memory for nonverbal material (Holmes, 1987).

Absence seizures, while not usually affecting memory, will have an impact on sustained attention. This deficit appears to occur both during and between seizures. Again, medications, particularly barbiturates and benzodiazepines, may adversely affect attention span (Holmes, 1987).

Behaviors

The relationship of epilepsy to behavioral disturbances has provoked much controversy. There has been great debate among authors as to whether or not seizures can be linked to specific psychological or behavioral disorders. This debate will likely continue for some time. But behavioral changes, as a result of brain dysfunction, medication side effects, personal, family or social stresses, anxiety, or depression that affect an individual's ability to function in society all impact the occupational therapy treatment program. Some common behavior patterns may become evident to the therapist during treatment. Other behaviors may be more subtle, or may be confused with psychopathological states.

Hallucinations, particularly olfactory hallucinations, are fairly common with seizures. The hallucination usually takes the form of an unpleasant odor. Visual hallucinations may occur when there is a focus in the right temporal lobe.

Seizures arising in or propagating to the reticular formation may produce unconsciousness (Sands, 1982). Some individuals will have altered states of consciousness as part of the seizure, or as the sole manifestation of the seizure. In these states, the individual is not unconscious, but is unaware of his or her surroundings and may behave in a purposeful, albeit inappropriate manner.

Seizures arising in the medial temporal structures may result in an amnesia. A right temporal lobe focus may result in a feeling of familiarity or unfamiliarity (a deja vu or jamais vu experience). These individuals sometimes complain of poor memory or a feeling that their thought processes have been forcibly stopped.

Some automatisms that are part of a seizure, or that occur just after a seizure, include motor activity such as picking or disrobing. The activity appears purposeful and deliberate but is actually a part of the ictal disturbance.

Feeling states are common with seizure disorders. Sensations of ecstasy, fear or dread are commonly reported with seizures. Sudden bursts of laughter may also be the result of a seizure disorder.

In addition to these ictal disturbances of epilepsy, personality problems, social adjustment difficulties, conflicts (conscious and unconscious) and the struggle to cope with the tasks of independent living all may give rise to tension and stress in persons with epilepsy. Anxiety and emotional stress that arise out of these difficulties without the individual's awareness of their precise nature are known to increase the frequency of seizures (Sands, 1982).

Sands (1982) cites several factors involved in the adjustment to seizure disorders. These include: the individual's acceptance of and adjustment to the seizure disorder and the medical regimen necessary to control the disorder, the individual's understanding and accommodation to the behaviors that are a result of the seizure, the individual's ability to adjust to the emotional stresses of having epilepsy, the individual's ability to cope with the demands of independent living and social interaction, and the individual's ability to deal with the prejudices and barriers of social response to the disorder.

Like many other medical disorders, epilepsy is both an individual medical disorder and a family problem. Whatever the age of seizure onset, most individuals and their families have increased anxiety with the first seizure. This new anxiety will change their lives. If seizure onset is at an early age, the child and family must adapt to the epilepsy while dealing with the normal developmental process. Because of the fear of injury associated with seizures, there appears to be a higher incidence of dependency in children with epilepsy than is found in children with other chronic diseases such as diabetes or cystic fibrosis (Holmes, 1987).

Some children who lose consciousness during seizures must rely on observers for their impression of behaviors during and after seizures. Their self image is frequently based on these subjective opinions of others. Additional burdens for children with epilepsy are the associated motor impairments and learning disabilities discussed earlier. These deficits may further complicate the child's ability to solve problems and compete physically and academically with his/her peers.

Couple these problems with the tendency for overprotectiveness on the part of the family and the cycle of fear, loss of control, inability to perform, lack of self esteem, and dependency begins. The therapist who works with children with epilepsy must be willing to spend considerable time with the child's parents, discussing behavior modification, epilepsy education, safe and independent activities of daily living and potential educational or vocational problems.

Seizure characteristics themselves have the potential to create behavior problems. Although an aura may give an individual sufficient warning of an impending seizure, allowing the opportunity to move to a safe place or secure area, the aura may be the actual onset of the seizure and may cause fear rather than comfort. Some individuals may cry out at the onset of their seizures, startling others in the room. Some individuals cannot respond to questions and may appear defiant to the questioner. Automatisms may be frightening or appear bizarre to those who do not understand their implications. And the individual may be confused, fatigued, sleepy or even incontinent as a result of seizure activity.

There is a direct correlation between seizure frequency and seizure control and the adjustment to normal daily living tasks. The time and place of seizure occurrence can impact on the individual's adjustment efforts. As noted by Santilli and Sierzant (1987), some anticonvulsant drugs also impact on behaviors (see Figure 4).

"The multiply disabled person with epilepsy has a more difficult task in coping and adjusting. The total disability is more than the mere sum of the two or more disabling conditions. Seizures and cognitive deficits due to brain damage, depending upon degree of impairment, present a different order of adjustment problems than do seizures and a hemiplegia or seizures and an orthopedic disabil-

FIGURE 4. Anticonvulsant Medications — Adapted from Santilli and Sierzant (1987)

Generic Name	Trade Name	Therapeutic Dosage	Therapeutic Drug Blood Level	Seizure Type	Common Side Effects
Carbamazepine	Tegretol	10–15 mg/kg/day Half-life: 9–19 hrs	4–12 µg/ml	Secondary tonic-clonic Complex partial Simple partial	Lethargy Dizziness Ataxia, behavioral changes Blurred vision Aplastic anemia Double vision
Clonazepam	Clonopin	0.05–0.2 mg/kg/day Half-life: 18–20 hrs	20–80 µg/ml	Absence Myoclonic	Drowsiness, slurred speech Double vision, behavior changes, increased salivation
Divaloroex sodium Valproate Acid	Depakote Depakene	20–60 mg/kg/day Half-life: 6–18 hrs	50–100 µg/ml	Myoclonic Absence, tonic-clonic Mixed seizure types	Hair loss, tremor Elevated liver enzymes Irregular menses Increased appetite Nausea & vomiting (not as common with Depakote)

Drug	Brand	Dosage / Half-life	Therapeutic Level	Seizure Type	Side Effects
Ethosuximide	Zarontin	15–35 mg/kg/day Half-life: 24–72 hrs	40–100 µg/ml	Absence	GI upset Loss of appetite Headache, lethargy Behavior changes Dizziness
Phenobarbital	Luminal	4–6 mg/kg/day Half-life: 53–104 hrs	10–40 µg/ml	Tonic-clonic Partial seizures	Changes in sleep pattern Drowsiness, excitability Irritability Cognitive impairment
Phenytoin	Dilantin	5–10 mg/kg/day Half-life: 7–22 hrs	10–25 µg/ml	Tonic-clonic Complex partial Simple partial	Nystagmus Blurred vision Double vision Gingival hyperplasia Ataxia, skin rash Folate deficiency
Primidone	Mysoline	12–25 mg/kg/day Half-life: 3–12 hrs	5–12 µg/ml	Tonic-clonic Complex partial Simple partial	Drowsiness Hyperactivity in children Ataxia Behavior changes

ity. Attitudes — especially those of self-worth, self-esteem and confidence — become differentially exacerbated in the multiply disabled individual with epilepsy" (Sands, 1982).

Vocational Adjustment

Several obvious problems face the individual with seizures when preparing to enter or continue in the job market. If the individual has concomitant associated difficulties, additional handicapping conditions may present themselves.

One of the most difficult problems to confront the individual with epilepsy is the lack of understanding and the subsequent fear of employers to hire the individual with a seizure disorder. The Epilepsy Foundation of America indicates that the unemployment rate for persons with seizures is twice the national average (Sands, 1982).

Factors affecting the employment of individuals with epilepsy include seizure control, seizure frequency, seizure prodrome, and seizure type. Stress, in relation to vocational activity, is another factor that may affect employability.

Employers frequently seek full medical control of the seizure activity before making a full employment offer. It is important for the occupational therapist to help educate employers about the employability of persons with epilepsy. It is generally accepted that about 80% of those with epilepsy are competitively employable (Sands, 1982). It is critical that the occupational therapist assist the person with epilepsy to objectively look at skills, abilities, and limitations when approaching the job market. Helping the individual to look at all the factors affecting vocational choices will prevent an inability to answer the difficult questions of the employer. And, as discussed regarding safety measures in Activities of Daily Living, the therapist can assist the person with epilepsy to carefully examine how a job may be done safely and effectively.

Aptitude, achievement capabilities, memory, ability to attend to task, personal work skills, and interests play a part in vocational evaluation for the individual with seizures as it does for any other individual. The complete evaluation of the activities and responses both during and after the seizure will help the therapist and the seizure-prone individual to understand what precautions may be necessary at the job site, what education needs to be done with colleagues and co-workers, and what medical information needs to be readily available on the job. Other considerations at the job site include the identification of any precipitants of seizures, if applicable. Alerting co-workers to consistent auras, and suggesting actions to take when they observe that aura, may be helpful to prevent fear and injury on the job. An employer needs to understand what, if any, recovery time is needed for the employee following the seizure.

It is important that an individual with seizures communicate with his or her employer regarding the disorder. "If individuals are accepting of their current seizure status, the person with whom they are interacting tends to be more at ease in relation to the condition. When a person can comfortably and succinctly discuss epilepsy with an employment interviewer, the interviewer becomes more assured that medical status will be understandable to the line supervisor. If counselor (therapist) and client can successfully work toward the client's acceptance of the disability, the client is better prepared to modify the uncertainties and negative attitudes that are encountered in the social, educational, and vocational arenas" (Sands, 1982).

CONCLUSION

The role of the occupational therapist with epilepsy is complex and varied, and spans many areas of professional expertise. It is a fallacy for occupational therapists to believe that they will never work with individuals having seizure disorders. With 1% of the U.S. population having epilepsy, it is likely that the therapist will not only work with seizure-prone individuals in the treatment setting, but will have contact with people with seizures in all walks of life.

Epilepsy is a brain disorder that impacts the physical, social, emotional, educational, recreational, and vocational functioning of all who are affected by it. The treatment of epilepsy is a challenging and rewarding practice area for occupational therapists, and our impact on treatment is just beginning to be recognized and developed.

REFERENCES

1. Black, R., Hermann, B., & Shope, J. (1982). *Nursing management of epilepsy*. Maryland: Aspen System Corporation.

2. Day, S. (1984). Occupational therapy assessment and treatment in a hospital setting for patients with epilepsy. *Occupational Therapy in Health Care*, Summer, 53-62.

3. Dreifuss, F. (1983): *Pediatric epileptology*. Massachusetts: John Wright.

4. Epilepsy Foundation of America, 4351 Garden City Drive, Landover, Maryland, 20785, (301) 459-3700. Personal communication (1988).

5. Holmes, G. (1987). *Diagnosis and management of seizures in children*. Pennsylvania: W.B. Saunders.

6. Pedley, T. & Meldrum, B. (eds.). (1985). *Recent advances in epilepsy*. New York: Churchill Livingston.

7. Sands, H. (ed.).(1982). *Epilepsy-A handbook for the mental health professional*. New York: Brunner/Mazel.

8. Santilli, N. (1987). Epilepsy: Care of the child and family. *Pediatric Nursing Forum, 2*(3).

9. Santilli, N., & Sierzant, T. (1987). Advances in the treatment of epilepsy. *Journal of Neuroscience Nursing, 19*(3), 141-155.

Early Intervention:
New Directions
for Occupational Therapists

Roseann C. Schaaf, MED, OTR/L
Laura N. Gitlin, PhD

SUMMARY. This paper provides an overview of the critical need for early intervention services, the specific role of occupational therapists in early intervention settings, and the training implications for the preparation of occupational therapists with expanded roles, responsibilities and skills. An intervention approach that is multidisciplinary, culturally relevant, and family centered in nature is proposed as one way of redefining the occupational therapist's contribution and strategy in early intervention settings. Recommendations are presented regarding the education and preparation of occupational therapists for their new directions in early intervention and the potential increase in demands for their services.

INTRODUCTION

Newborns, infants and toddlers diagnosed as developmentally at high risk now have a greater chance of survival than ever before due to the dramatic advances in medical technology (Mitchell, 1985; Weiner and Koppelman, 1987). The substantial increase in the

Roseann Schaaf is an instructor in the Department of Occupational Therapy at Thomas Jefferson University and also maintains a private practice in pediatrics. Address correspondence to 130 S. 9th Street, Suite 820, Department of Occupational Therapy, Philadelphia, PA 19107. Laura N. Gitlin is an assistant professor in the Department of Occupational Therapy at Thomas Jefferson University and is a research sociologist.

75

number of infants and toddlers surviving with developmental delays or disabilities has created a dramatic new need for a greater number of special services and more qualified personnel to deliver the breadth of interventions required by these children (Weiner and Koppelman, 1987). The broad range of service needs handicapped children in the zero to three age range population require, coupled with new federal incentives to develop alternative treatment models, challenges the field of occupational therapy to expand traditional roles and models of care.

The recent passage of the Education of the Handicapped Act Amendments of 1986 (Public Law 99-457) includes several unique aspects which will influence occupational therapy service delivery in early intervention. First, the law mandates the provision of comprehensive, community-based services to infants and toddlers with handicaps and their families (AOTA, 1986a). Second, the law emphasizes the involvement of parents and/or caregivers in the intervention process. Third, occupational therapy is identified as a primary early intervention service rather than a related service under the auspices of special education.

The redefinition of the role of occupational therapy and the provision of services to families on the community level, as delineated in this law, will have immediate and long-term implications for the number of therapists needed and the nature of their training in the field of newborn and infant rehabilitation (Weiner and Koppelman, 1987; personal communication, Barbara Hanft, November 11, 1987, AOTA, 1986a).

This paper provides an overview of the critical need for early intervention services, the specific role of occupational therapists in early intervention settings, and the training implications for the preparation of occupational therapists with expanded roles, responsibilities and skills. An intervention approach that is multidisciplinary, culturally relevant, and family centered in nature is proposed as one way of redefining the occupational therapist's contribution and strategy in early intervention settings. This information is presented in order to educate and prepare therapists regarding new directions for occupational therapy in early intervention and the potential increase in demands for their services.

THE NEED FOR EARLY INTERVENTION

There is growing empirical evidence that neonates, infants and toddlers who are either environmentally, biologically or medically at risk, developmentally delayed and/or handicapped derive innumerable short and long-term benefits from the early identification of the problem and the implementation of an appropriate intervention strategy. Studies from diverse fields, such as education, rehabilitation and pediatrics, and ranging in methodological sophistication and soundness, have strongly supported the efficacy of an early intervention model for disabled children ranging in age from zero to three (Shonkoff and Hauser-Cram, 1987; Meisels, 1985; Ramey, Bryant, Sparling, and Wasik, 1985; Hanson, 1985; Guralnick and Bricker, 1985; Reynolds, Egan, and Lerner, 1983; Als, Lawton, Brown, Giber, Duffy,, McAnulty, and Blickman, 1986; Subramanian, Clark-Prakash, Dadina, Ferrara and Johnson, 1986; Ottenbacher and Petersen, 1985; Palti-Hava, 1984; Ramey and Campbell, 1984; Greenspan and White, 1985).

Specifically, evaluations of early intervention programs varying in type of services and interventions have reported statistically significant developmental gains for the zero to three groups in motor skills, social-emotional level, language ability, and cognitive domains that are essential prerequisites to academic behaviors (Resnick, Eyler, Nelson, Eitzman and Bucciarelli, 1987). Research evidence from studies on school aged children suggest that potential problems in the school age years may be averted by the identification of the handicapping condition in neonates and infants and the early implementation of a treatment program well before the child enters school (Sell, Gaines, Gluckman and Williams, 1985; Brazelton, 1982; Dalton, 1973, Greenspan, 1981).

Studies evaluating the specific contribution of occupational therapy treatment modalities in early intervention programs have also demonstrated benefits in the areas of fine, gross, sensory, visual, motor and self-help skills (Hourcade and Parette, 1986; Bailey and Bricker, 1985; Oelwein, Fewell and Pruess, 1985; Chestnut, 1977; Zausmer, 1972; Resnick, et al., 1987; Campbell, 1985; Piper, Mazer, Hardy, and Doucette, 1986; Brazelton, 1982; Ottenbacher, Muller, Brandt and Heintzelman, 1987; Russman, 1986).

Family Centered Intervention

In addition to support for the efficacy of early intervention services for the child, there is growing research evidence regarding the benefit and need for a family centered intervention approach. Early infant assessment and treatment have been shown to have many positive benefits for family and caregivers. The data indicate that the inclusion of parents in a treatment program tends to decrease parental anxiety and stress. A family centered approach appears to produce significant positive behavioral changes in both the parent and the child (Leander and Pettett, 1986; Salitros, 1986; Hanson, 1985; Consolvo, 1986; Censullo, 1986; Wasserman, Inui, Barriatua, Carter and Lippincott, 1984; Weiner and Koppelman, 1987; Meisels, 1985; Bryant and Ramey, 1984; Allen, Affleck, McGrade and McQueeney, 1984; Kysela and Marfo, 1983; Macy, Solomon, Schoen and Galey, 1983; Russman, 1986; Moran, 1985).

Interventions which include the family or caregiver have also been shown to be more effective in promoting developmental gains in the infant due to continued contact and reinforcement of the intervention strategy by family members (Allen et al., 1984). Occupational therapy approaches which involve training parents in the areas of positioning, feeding, handling and enriching the sensory environment, have been shown to be effective interventions in the home environment (Campbell, 1985; Brazelton, 1982; Russman, 1986). However, more research is needed to explore the influence of specific interventions on the parent-child relationship and to examine how treatment promotes adaptive development.

Previous research on mother-child interaction patterns in families without disability has clearly indicated the relationship of the infant's development to parental responsiveness and, in turn, the effect of parental behavior on subsequent development (Lewis, and Coates, 1980; Jaskir and Lewis, 1981). The evidence from studies comparing interaction patterns in normal and atypical families suggests that mothers of at-risk and developmentally delayed children, as a group, need professional support and assistance which is most effectively provided in the context of an early intervention program (Kysela and Marfo, 1983). In light of this body of literature, it is essential that effective early intervention approaches incorporate the family and caregiver in the evaluation, treatment and planning process.

Cultural Implications

There is substantive data documenting that infants and children from impoverished environments are at greater risk for developmental delays (Hobel, 1985; Hutchins, Placek and Walker, 1983). However, it is this very group which has been the most difficult to service adequately because traditional intervention approaches have been insensitive to sociocultural differences in parenting styles, attitudes, social supports and resources (Allen et al., 1984).

The early intervention literature indicates that for interventions to be meaningful and effective, programming must be family-specific, and capture the cultural diversity and specific environmental concerns of each family serviced (Allen et al., 1984; Kysela and Marfo 1983). Professionals must be skilled in adapting state-of-the-art intervention techniques which enhance parental involvement in the treatment process and assure continued developmental benefit for the child and family from diverse cultural and socio-economic backgrounds.

PERSONNEL NEEDS IN THE EARLY
INTERVENTION SETTING

The evidence supporting early intervention programs helped pave the way for a federal mandate of an array of services to both handicapped children aged 0-5 and their families. The passage of Public Law 99-457 has thus created a critical demand for additional personnel and specifically for occupational therapists trained in the provision of early intervention services and capable of functioning in a variety of capacities and diverse settings. National, state and local surveys conducted to assess personnel needs following the implementation of Public Law 99-457 have affirmed the need for more staffing and have projected critical shortages of trained professionals in the future (McLaughlin, Smith-Davis and Burke, 1986). Occupational therapists need to be aware of these potential shortages, the increased demands for their services, and the context in which early intervention will be practiced.

National Needs

In a 1986 national survey, Weiner and Koppelman (1987), found that nearly 90% of states reported a lack of sufficient personnel, including occupational therapists, to serve school-aged handicapped children. Another national survey by Meisels, Harbin, Modigliani and Olson, (1986) indicated that 96% of all states reported a shortage of personnel, including physical therapists, speech therapists, and occupational therapists, to service children aged zero to three. Furthermore, 83% of the states expected the shortages to continue through 1989.

The results of a recent survey conducted by the American Occupational Therapy Association (AOTA), indicated that 70% of occupational therapy program directors and state representatives to AOTA had difficulty recruiting qualified occupational therapists to fill pediatric positions in their states (Henderson, Lawlor and Pehoski, 1986). Additionally, 45% of the respondents believed that staffing shortages were due to the lack of appropriately trained therapists in the early intervention field and to a shortage of therapists in general. The data suggest that the need for occupational therapists will sharply increase in the next few years, aggravating an already acute shortage of qualified therapists with the necessary expertise in early intervention. Furthermore, according to state estimates from AOTA, occupational therapists with expertise in pediatrics and early intervention will be in great demand nationwide (personal communication, Hanft, November 11, 1987).

Available data on national employment patterns of occupational therapists suggest that therapists overwhelmingly continue to select employment in institutional environments based on a medical model of service delivery as opposed to seeking employment in the community-based health care system (AOTA, 1985). Reasons cited for this imbalance include inadequate educational preparation for work within non-traditional systems, inadequate preparation for work with specialty populations, lack of supervision in community environments, and lower pay scales. This employment pattern has serious implications for the delivery of early intervention services in light of PUBLIC LAW 99-457 which mandates the development of community-based programs.

State Needs

Similar shortages and demands exist at state and local levels. For example, the Pennsylvania Department of Education describes an acute need for a greater number of and more highly qualified occupational therapists to service all exceptional children (Comprehensive System of Personnel Development Needs Survey, 1987). Additionally, the Pennsylvania Bureau of Special Education conducted a state wide survey in 1986 to identify strength and needs of programs in Pennsylvania for children with handicaps between zero to three years of age. Approximately 626 parents, professionals and administrators responded to the survey. Of the 25 listed services, "Occupational Therapy was perceived state-wide as the third greatest need behind transportation and specialized day care" (personal communication, Dr. Makuch, Director, Bureau of Special Education, January, 1988).

Local Needs

To fully understand the scope of need for occupational therapists trained in early intervention, the authors conducted a telephone survey of the 16 major community-based early intervention programs in Philadelphia County. Since little is known about the particular staffing patterns and needs of non-institutional environments, and in keeping with the specifications of Public Law 99-457, only community-based centers were surveyed to assess the roles of occupational therapists in these settings.

The survey indicated that all 16 facilities provided a variety of services to the zero to three population including several types of occupational therapy services (e.g., sensory stimulation, motor development, parent education, adaptive equipment, handling and consultation). Occupational and Speech therapists were present in every facility on a part or full-time basis in contrast to other early intervention team professionals who were not uniformly represented in each agency. The presence of a part or full time occupational therapist in each facility and the diverse services they provided underscores the key role of the profession in the provision of early intervention services.

The survey also highlighted the discrepancy between service needs and actual provision of occupation therapy. Only 21% of the projected occupational therapy service hours needed by children were met in the 16 centers. Furthermore, 60% of the facilities surveyed reported difficulty filling vacant positions by qualified occupational therapists. Fifty-five percent indicated that therapists often lacked direct experience with the zero to three population or lacked training in such necessary skills as consultation, working with families, teachers, small groups, handling infants or knowledge of team-care approaches. The shortage of trained personnel is dramatized by the fact that ninety percent of the agencies project a critical need to substantially increase occupational therapy hours over the next five years.

AN INTERVENTION APPROACH
FOR OCCUPATIONAL THERAPISTS

Training Needs

The local, state and national data on personnel needs clearly indicates the necessity to educate and train additional therapists with specific skills in early intervention. Practice approaches which address community-based settings, team-care, and family-based treatment models are also needed.

Traditionally, occupational therapists have served neonates, infants and toddlers in institutional settings using a direct service model based primarily on a medical model of care. The focus on individual disability, with minimal consideration of the role of family and environment on adaptive behavior, has limited the scope and function of occupational therapy in the intervention process, (Brazelton, 1982; Anderson, 1986; AOTA, 1986a).

In light of recent legislative changes and the growing demand for occupational therapy services, the American Occupational Therapy Association has reevaluated the role of practice in early intervention. It has also underlined the importance of training that goes beyond skill development in individual assessment and treatment approaches to an examination of the socio-cultural, environmental context of individual functioning (AOTA, 1986c). AOTA has defined occupational therapy in early intervention in the following manner.

"Occupational therapy personnel use purposeful activity in the development or restoration of function to help the child and family develop resources to meet personal needs and the demands of the environment. The child's occupations of movement, play, eating, interacting with others, dressing, bathing and the like are the purposeful activities used in early childhood intervention to promote normal development and adaptive coping behaviors. Treatment stems from a scientifically based neurophysiological framework. Services are provided to help parents in their roles as providers and primary caregivers. Treatment may be provided in collaboration with other disciplines and professionals . . . Occupational therapy in early intervention promotes independent function and adaptive interaction with the environment through the use of age appropriate, purposeful activity."

Training Recommendations

The shift in role definition highlights the need for an adequate knowledge base in family systems, educational systems and community resources as essential for effective short and long-term service delivery approaches for children with handicaps. The "Essentials of Entry-Level Education in Occupational Therapy" (AOTA, 1983) require knowledge and skill in generalized practice. However, advanced knowledge of leadership, managerial, consultative and technical skills required for treating newborns, infants and toddlers in an environmental context have not traditionally been a part of the undergraduate curriculum (Anderson, 1986; Henderson et al., 1986; Hanft, personal communication, 1987; AOTA, 1986b; AOTA, 1986c).

Recommendations to improve occupational therapy education in the areas of pediatrics include the following:

1. the development of graduate level studies with a specialization tract or certification program, (Henderson et al., 1986; AOTA, 1986b; AOTA, 1986c);
2. the introduction of curricula on family systems and care providers;
3. theory and theory-based assessments, specialty practice much as sensory integration and neurodevelopmental treatment, exposure to the variety of service delivery models, and evaluation techniques of these models;
4. knowledge of and experience with the variety of roles of the occupational therapist working with a multidisciplinary team, (Henderson et al., 1986; Hanft, personal communication, 1987).

Findings from the Philadelphia County survey also illustrate the need for occupational therapists to move beyond traditional intervention approaches to meet the changing demands of the early intervention system. Three themes emerge from the interviews with directors of the community-based programs:

1. the need for therapists to work in a consultative and collaborative structure with families, teachers and other persons involved with the child;
2. the need for therapists to be skilled in small group processes in order to communicate across disciplines and function effectively on a team;
3. and the need for therapists to actively consider and incorporate the individual's family, environment and culture in the assessment, treatment and planning process.

These three points are also emphasized in Public Law 99-457 which, as discussed previously, has mandated the inclusion of parents or primary caregivers in the intervention process.

In light of the early intervention literature, documented personnel needs and federal legislation, there is an urgent need for occupational therapists to redefine their role in early intervention and move from traditional, direct service models to a family centered, environmentally oriented, multidisciplinary approach in the assessment and treatment process. Occupational therapists must be prepared to understand the individual infant's needs in the context of the specific environmental concerns of the family's lifestyle and culture if the profession is to emerge as a leader in the delivery of early intervention services. The expansion of the therapist's traditional role to include problem-solving in any environmental context, and consultation, and collaboration in complex delivery organizations, will assure efficient and effective approaches to the delivery of services. A consultative, collaborative approach to care will also impact a greater number of consumers. The proposed training recommendations specify the need for therapists with advanced knowledge, skill and leadership ability to function effectively in a comprehensive and community-based model of service provision.

CONCLUSION

This paper identifies the changing trends in early intervention and the new roles occupational therapists will have in community-based care settings. It is suggested that advanced training of therapists is needed for occupational therapists to function effectively.

Training which focuses on family dynamics and team-care approaches will have direct benefit on the: 1) quality and type of services provided to newborns and infants with handicaps; 2) quality and range of occupational therapeutic services to family and other caregivers; 3) role and functioning of the occupational therapist on the early intervention team, and 4) consequently the effectiveness and efficiency of the entire intervention process. It is through a multidisciplinary, family-centered, culturally relevant approach to care that occupational therapists will be best prepared to meet the challenge and demand for services created by new federal legislation.

REFERENCES

American Occupational Therapy Association (1983). Guide to Compliance with the 1983 Essentials for an Educational Program for the Occupational Therapist: Rockville, MD.

American Occupational Therapy Association (1985). *Occupational Therapy Manpower: A Plan for Progress*.

American Occupational Therapy Association (1986a). Government and Legal Affairs Division Bulletin: Rockville, MD: American Occupational Therapy Association.

American Occupational Therapy Association (1986b). Early childhood intervention (Position Paper) *American Journal of Occupational Therapy*, *40*(12), 833-4.

American Occupational Therapy Association (1986c). Roles and functions of occupational therapy in early childhood intervention (Position Paper) *American Journal of Occupational Therapy*, *40*(12), 835-8.

Als, H., Lawton, G., Brown, E., Giber R., Duffy, E.H., McAnulty, G., Blickman, J.G. (1986). Individualized behavioral and environmental care for the very low birth weight preterm infant at high risk for bronchopulmonary dysplasia: Neonatal intensive care unit and development outcome. *Pediatrics*, *78*(6), 1123-32.

Allen, D.A., Affleck, G., McGrade, B.J., McQueeney, M. (1984). Fac,tors in the effectiveness of early childhood intervention for low socioeconomic status families. *Education and Training of the Mentally Retarded*, *19*(4), 254-260.

Anderson, J. (1986). Sensory intervention with the preterm infant in the neonatal intensive care unit. *American Journal of Occupational Therapy*, *40*(10), 19-26.

Bailey, E.J. and Bricker, D. (1985). Evaluation of a three year early intervention demonstration project. *Topics in Early Childhood Special Education*, *5*(2), 52-65.

Brazelton, T.B. (1982). Early Intervention: What does it mean? *Theory and Research in Behavioral Pediatrics*, Vol 1. New York: Plenum Publishing Corp.

Bryant, D.M. and Ramey, C.T. (1984). Prevention-oriented infant education programs. Special Issue: Infant Intervention Programs: Truths and Untruths. *Journal of Children in Contemporary Society*, *17*(1), 17-35.

Campbell, S.K. (1985). Effects of developmental intervention in the special care nursery. *The Advances in Developmental and Behavioral Pediatrics*, Greenwich, CT: JAI Press.

Censullo, M. (1986). Home care of the high-risk newborn. *Journal of Obstetrics and Gynecological Neonatal Nursing*, *15*(2), 146-153.

Chestnut, J.M., (1977). *Early infant intervention program: The effect on the developmentally delayed infants.*

Consolvo, C.A. (1986). Relieving parental anxiety in the care-by-parent unit. *Journal of Obstetrics and Gynecological Neonatal Nursing*, *15*(2), 154-159.

Dalton, M.E. (1973). "Who shall begin? What difference does It make? Early childhood intervention." *Pediatric Annals*, 66-91.

Greenspan, S.I., White, K.R. (1985). The efficacy of preventive intervention: A glass half full? *Zero to Three*, *5*(4), 1-5.

Greenspan, S.I., (1981). *Psychopathology and Adaptation in Infancy and Early Childhood: Principles of Clinical Diagnosis and Preventive Intervention*, New York: International Universities Press.

Guralnick, M. and Bricker, D. (1986). The effectiveness of early intervention for children with cognitive and general developmental delays. *The Effectiveness of Early Intervention*, New York: Academic Press.

Hanson, M.J. (1985). An analysis of the effects of early intervention services for infants and toddlers with moderate and severe handicaps. *Topics in Early Childhood Special Education*, 5(2), 36-51.

Henderson, A., Lawlor, M. and Pehoski, C. (1986). *Proceedings of the Maternal and Child Health*. Boston University pediatric occupational therapy symposium sponsored by the Division of Maternal and Child Health Bureau of Health Care Resources and Services Administration Public Health Service.

Hobel, Calvin J., (1985). Factors before pregnancy that influence brain development in *Prenatal and Perinatal Factors Associated with Brain Disorders*. U.S. Dept. of HHS, NIH Publication #85-1149.

Hourcade, J.J., Parette, H.P. (1986). Early intervention programming: Correlates of progress. *Perceptual and Motor Skills*, 62(1), 58.

Hutchins, V., Placek, P., Walker, A. (1983). Trend in maternal and infant health factors associated with low infant birth weight. United States 1972 & 1980. Preliminary results presented October 17, 1983 to the Institute of Medicine.

Jaskir, J. and Lewis, M. (1981). A Factor analytic study of mother-infant interaction at 3, 12, and 24 months. Presented at the annual meeting of the Eastern Psychological Association, New York.

Kysela, G.M. and Marfo, K. (1983). Mother-child interactions and early intervention programs for handicapped infants and young children. *Educational Psychology* 3(3-4), 201-212.

Leander, D., Pettett, G. (1986). Parental response to the birth of a high-risk neonatal: Dynamics and management. *Physical and Occupational Therapy in Pediatrics*, 6(3-4), 205-216.

Lewis, M. and Coates, D.L. (1980). Mother-infant interactions and cognitive development in twelve week-old infants. *Infant Behavior Development*, 3, 95-105.

Macy, D.J., Solomon, G.S., Schoen, M., Galey, G.S. (1983). The debt project: Early intervention for handicapped children and their parents. *Exceptional Children*, 49(5), 447-448.

McLaughlin, M., Smith-Davis, J. and Burke, P. (1986). *Personnel to Educate the Handicapped*: College Park, MD: Institute for the Study of Exceptional Children and Youth, Dept. of Special Education, College of Education, University of MD.

Meisels, S.J., (1985) The efficacy of early intervention: Why are we still asking this question? *Topics in Early Childhood Special Education*, 5(2), 1-11.

Meisels, S.J., Harbin, G., Modigliani, K., Olson, K., (1986). Formulating optimal state early childhood intervention policies. Paper presented at CEC Conference, Louisville, KT.

Mitchell, R.G. (1985). *Objectives and Outcomes of Perinatal Care*. Lancet, 2(8461), 931-4.

Moran, M. (1985). Families in early intervention: Effects of program variables. *Zero to Three, 5*(5), 11-14.

Oelwein, P.L., Fewell, R.R., Pruess, J.B. (1985). The efficacy of intervention at outreach sites of the program for children with down syndrome and other developmental delays. *Topics in Early Childhood Special Education, 5*(2), 78-87.

Ottenbacher, K.J., Muller, L., Brandt, D., Heintzelman, A., (1987). The effectiveness of tactile stimulation as a form of early intervention: A quantitative evaluation. *Journal of Developmental and Behavioral Pediatrics, 8*(2), 68-76.

Ottenbacher, K.J. and Petersen, P. (1985). The efficacy of early intervention programs for children with organic impairment: A quantitative review. *Evaluation and Program Planning, 8*(2), 135-146.

Palti-Hava, (1984). Children's home environments: Comparison of a group exposed to a stimulation intervention program with controls. *Early Child Development and Care, 13*(2), 193-212.

Piper, M., Mazer, B., Hardy, S., Doucette, C. (1986). Monitoring the effects of early physical therapy on the high-risk infant: Preliminary results. *Physical and Occupational Therapy in Pediatrics, 6*(3), 1-4.

Ramey, C., Bryan, D., Sparling, J., Wasik, B. (1985). Project Care: A comparison of two early intervention strategies to prevent retarded development. *Topics in Early Childhood Special Education, 5*(2), 12-25.

Ramey, C.T. and Campbell, F.A. (1984). Preventive education for high-risk children: Cognitive consequences of the Carolina Abecedarian Project. *American Journal of Mental Deficiency, 88*(5), 515-523.

Resnick, M.B., Eyler, F.D., Nelson, R.M., Eitzman, D.V., Bucciarelli, R.L. (1987). Developmental intervention for low birth weight infants: Improved early developmental outcome. *Pediatrics, 80*(1), 68-74.

Reynolds, L., Egan, R., Lerner, J. (1983). Efficacy of early intervention on pre-academic deficits: A review of the literature. *Topics in Early Childhood Special Education, 3*(3), 47-55.

Russman, B.S. (1986). Are infant stimulation programs useful? *Archives of Neurology, 43*(3), 282-283.

Salitros, P.H. (1986). Transitional infant care: A bridge to home for high-risk infants. *Neonatal Network, 4*(4), 35-41.

Sell, E.J., Gaines, J.A., Gluckman, C., Williams, E. (1985). Early identification of learning problems in neonatal intensive care graduates. *American Journal of Disabled Children, 139*(5), 460-463.

Shonkoff, J.P., Hauser-Crain, P. (1987). Early intervention for disabled infants and their families: A quantitative analysis. *Pediatrics, 80*(5), 650-658.

Subramanian, C., Clark-Prakash, C., Dadina, Z.K., Ferrara, B., Johnson, D.E. (1986). Intensive care for high-risk infants in Calcutta—Efficacy and cost. *American Journal of Disabled Children, 140*(9), 885-888.

Wasserman, R.C., Inui, T.S., Barriatua, R.D., Carter, W.B., Lippincott, P. (1984). Pediatric clinician's support for parents makes a difference: An outcome based analysis of clinician-parent interaction. *Pediatrics*, 74(6), 1047-53.

Weiner, R., Koppelman, J. (1987). *Birth to 5: Serving the Youngest Handicapped Children*. Virginia: Capital Publications, Inc.

Zausmer, E., Pueschel, S.M., Shea, A. (1972). A sensory-motor stimulation program for the young child with Down's Syndrome. *MCH Exchange*, 2(4). An intervention program for Down's Syndrome at Boston Children's Hospital.

Occupational Therapy in a Regional Comprehensive Service System

David A. Ethridge, PhD, OTR, FAOTA
Peter Dimmer, MA, OTR
Beverly Harrison, BS, OTR
Denise Davis, BS, OTR

SUMMARY. This paper provides an overview of the diverse roles played by occupational therapists in a large regional comprehensive service system for persons with developmental disabilities. A brief description of the system is followed by a look at how occupational therapy services are provided within the regional center itself and a review of work training and day activities services as the service recipient moves toward greater independence and a lesser restrictive setting. In the community setting the occupational therapists roles are that of arranging for, monitoring and assuring delivery of appropriate services.

Occupational Therapy is a diverse profession. In a large regional comprehensive service system for persons with developmental disabilities the varied roles played by occupational therapists illustrates that diversity. All too often occupational therapists are cast as the crafts teacher in a classroom type setting where hospital residents produce trinkets and toys of generally inferior quality with little, if any, relationship shown between the activity and the reason for the hospital stay. Although such activity programs exist in many types

---

David A. Ethridge is Director of Oakdale Regional Center, Lapeer, MI 48446. Peter Dimmer is Director of Administrative-Clinical Support Services, Community Services Division, Oakdale Regional Center. Beverly Harrison is Chief of the Occupational Therapy Section, Oakdale Regional Center. Denise Davis is Day Services Program Liaison, Occupational Therapy Section, Oakdale Regional Center.

of facilities across the country they are considered diversional at best. They are not illustrative of the occupational therapy program in the comprehensive system described here.

To understand both the comprehensiveness of the system and the diversity of occupational therapy roles, this paper will present a brief description of the system, a look at how occupational therapy services are provided within the regional center itself, and a review of work training and day activities services which are arranged as the service recipient moves toward greater independence and a lesser restrictive setting. In the community setting the occupational therapists roles are that of arranging, monitoring, and assuring delivery of services to those who have moved into a community living arrangement. Occupational therapists are key members of the interdisciplinary team in all these settings.

OVERVIEW OF OAKDALE REGIONAL CENTER

Oakdale Regional Center (ORC) is a state residential facility for mentally retarded and developmentally disabled persons residing in five east-central counties in Michigan. The service region has a population of more than 825,000 persons. ORC, as the state-owned and operated regional facility, is an integral part of a comprehensive system of services which includes Community Mental Health programs administered by county boards, Intermediate School District special education services, and numerous other public and private agencies.

The mission of Oakdale Center has changed significantly since it opened in 1895 as a State Home for the Feebleminded and Epileptic with a capacity for 200 residents. This was Michigan's first institution to provide a state financed residence for handicapped persons where basic health care and living needs were met. It became a permanent home for many residents.

Changes in public attitudes during the 1960s resulted in new federal and state initiatives for education, training habilitation, care and community placement of developmentally handicapped persons which expedited the return of many residents to the community. Funding for special education and community services reduced the number of admissions to state facilities. Resident census at Oakdale

Center by mid-1984 was less than 500, a reduction of 3,900 (88%) in 28 years. It is currently 330.

The population in residence at ORC is one of persons with multi-handicaps and difficult management problems. Over 98% are above 18 years of age. Sixty-seven percent are profoundly retarded, and 21% are in the severe retardation range (less than 13% are mild to moderate). Forty-two percent also have a seizure disorder; 26% have cerebral palsy and nearly 50% are classified as having severe behavioral problems. Over 25% have visual impairments, and 12% have hearing impairments. Over 54% have four or more disabling conditions. The population in residence at the Center is the most severely disabled in the broad spectrum of persons with developmental disabilities.

In 1977 Oakdale Center was granted certification as an Intermediate Care Facility for the Mentally Retarded (ICF/MR), indicating compliance with state and federal standards in programs, staffing levels and residential structures. The Center currently holds two-year accreditation from The Accreditation Council On Services For People With Developmental Disabilities and has previously been reaccredited in 1984 and 1986.

As fully integrated community living has become the goal of all programs that serve persons with mental retardation and developmental disabilities, Oakdale Regional Center and the Community Mental Health (CMH) agencies have developed a comprehensive, integrated system of services in the region. In all operational aspects, Oakdale Regional Center is today an extended community service. State-county cooperation provides a continuum of care, treatment, training, and living opportunities for clients whether residing at the Center or in community homes. ORC and CMH programs are coordinated to avoid duplication of support services for mentally retarded persons residing in communities. Follow-up services for former ORC residents continue until local agencies assume full responsibility and/or independent living capability is assured.

Services are divided into two major categories: Residential Facility Services and Community Living Services. The Residential Facility Services are housed on a large central campus in which all the currently utilized facilities were totally remodeled in 1979-80 to meet existing regulations for Intermediate Care Facilities for Persons with Mental Retardation (ICF/MR) and to comply with Standards as established by the Accreditation Council On Services For People With Developmental Disabilities (ACDD). The Center has repeatedly received commendations for the design, excellence and efficiency of the facilities and programs from the various surveying bodies. The Community Living Services has offices on the main campus and operate primarily through contract facilities and programs for the 440 residents placed in the community settings. The resident population mirrors that of the Residential Facility with only a slightly lesser degree of impairment than noted above.

RESIDENTIAL FACILITY SERVICES

ORC operates on a decentralized unit plan utilizing an interdisciplinary team process. Units range in size from 20 to 100 residents based on physical plant accommodation and suitable groupings of residents. Staffing also varies in ratios due to both physical plant configuration and specific needs of the residents to be served.

Interdisciplinary Team Process

The interdisciplinary team process is an approach to evaluate, to diagnose and to develop an individual program plan in which professionals and paraprofessionals participate as a team. Each building or residential complex has an assigned group of professionals who make up the team but since each resident has unique needs the make-up of each team differs except for "care" members required by each team. The team focuses on identifying the developmental needs of the client and on devising ways to meet these needs. The interdisciplinary team participants all share information, recommendations and responsibility so that a unified and integrated habilitation program plan is developed. This approach differs greatly from the "multidisciplinary approach" in which representatives of each discipline view the client from their own perspectives reporting separately the findings and the recommendations each proposes to implement.

The "core" members of the interdisciplinary team includes the program director and/or assistant, physician, psychologist, occupational therapist, speech therapist, recreation therapist, nurse, dietitian, social worker, client and client's guardian. Based on client needs, additional staff who may attend team meetings as needed are the work evaluator, physical therapist, teacher, audiologist, dentist/assistant and community services personnel.

The occupational therapists are assigned to the residential units and interdisciplinary teams from a centralized occupational therapy services section which also supervises the work training program and provides liaison to community day programs. The occupational therapy services section is a part of the ORC Activities Therapy Department which also contains the speech therapy, physical therapy and recreational therapy services sections. The services of many of these sections are often interrelated and require close coordination to eliminate duplication and assure efficient utilization of resources. When applied in concert the result is a powerful cadre of skilled professionals dedicated to the assessment and provision of specialized services to the residents of ORC.

Assessments

The occupational therapist conducts assessments annually in conjunction with the client's yearly interdisciplinary team meeting for the purpose of developing a plan of service. As stated by Ellen Lederman

> the general purposes of occupational therapy evaluation of mentally retarded clients are:
> 1. to identify, define or diagnose problems which interfere with the acquisition of developmental skills or adaptive functioning;
> 2. to determine which problems may be partially ameliorated or totally resolved by occupational therapy intervention;
> 3. to establish a baseline of development, functioning and performance from which goals and objectives may be developed and treatment planned;
> 4. to establish a baseline of development, functioning, and performance to aid in determining at a later date the effec-

tiveness of occupational therapy intervention and the advis-
ability of continued intervention; and
5. to provide information for other disciplines. (Lederman,
1984)

The assessment, both unstructured and structured, involves observation which the therapist conducts. As there is no standardized
occupational therapy tool developed for evaluation of the mentally
retarded, tests from other disciplines such as psychology and education have been utilized. Areas evaluated are self-care tasks (eating,
dressing, and grooming), mobility, prevocational and vocational
abilities, play and leisure skills. Information from any staff member
(professional/paraprofessional) who may be familiar with the client
can be beneficial. The format utilized for these assessments is provided in Appendix 1.

An important part of the occupational therapy evaluation is determining the need for therapy.

Many factors need to be considered before making a final decision about the therapy needs of each individual. Among
these are the:

1. type of deficits or problems;
2. significance of the problem;
3. expected effectiveness of intervention;
4. type of program or treatment setting;
5. availability of other personnel. (ACDD, 1987)

The results of the assessment and recommendations are discussed
with the interdisciplinary team at the clients' annual team meeting.

Services

In general, the role of occupational therapy in an institution is
to aid the individual in achieving his or her maximum functional level in sensory, motor, perceptual, cognitive and social-emotional skills, as well as in activities of daily living.
The ultimate long term goal is to achieve the optimal level of
functioning and independence which will enable the individual
to leave the institution and live in a less restrictive setting or,

when this is not practical, to enable the individual to enjoy the highest possible quality of life within the institution. (Lederman, 1984)

A task-oriented approach is utilized to teach specific concrete skills utilizing a variety of activities and program media. The following list notes the various therapeutic activities which have been incorporated at ORC to enhance skill development:

1. sensory motor;
2. cognitive/perceptual motor;
3. activities of daily living (eating, dressing, grooming);
4. prevocational activity;
5. therapeutic arts and crafts;
6. woodworking;
7. horticulture and;
8. community awareness living activity.

For example, an individual may display limited functional hand skills without apparent neurological deficit. Assessment results indicate lack of motivation, refusal to participate and poor grasp. Implementation and treatment may involve various "team" members assigned to assist with simple fine motor grasp, release of objects and object placement tasks.

In addition to providing direct therapy services to the client, the therapist serves as a consultant for both professional and paraprofessional. Inservice training and ordering and maintenance of adaptive equipment are also important aspects of the occupational therapist's role.

Work Training and Day Activity

The Work Training Section at Oakdale Regional Center works in conjunction with Occupational Therapy Services. The Work Activities Program develops work stations, designs appropriate job duties and places residents in work situations developed to meet the resident's needs as defined in their plan of service. The work stations are generally, and at least initially, located in various settings within the facility although community based settings are used as appropriate and available. Providing the resident with the opportunity to experience work situations as similar to everyday employment as possible assists the resident in learning work patterns.

The Work Training Section at Oakdale Regional Center aims to assist the resident in the preparation for a more meaningful and productive life in a community setting. Employment assumes an important role in this. Oakdale Regional Center promotes the personal growth and development of the working resident as its primary concern rather than placing emphasis on production factors. A work experience provides residents the opportunity to develop and modify work habits, attitudes, self-concepts, motivation, and interpersonal relationships. Work makes a significant contribution to a resident's feeling of self work and importance. It leads to advancement towards community placement and a more independent life style.

Screenings, conducted by occupational therapy staff, provide valuable information regarding general condition, physical motor skills, activities of daily living skills, cognitive and perceptual motor skills, community living and socialization skills as well as the prevocational skills of the individual. This information is essential to the team discussions and decisions regarding progress and to fashion changes in the plan of service. From these screening and team discussions come the referrals for work training.

Upon receipt of a referral, a resident is scheduled to participate in a standardized vocational evaluation using the McCarron-Dial Work Evaluation System. A battery of tasks is utilized to obtain scores in the areas of verbal, sensory and fine/gross motor abilities and emotional adjustment. Vocational competency levels (such as day care, work activity, extended training, transitional placement) are determined for each of these factors. Test results can provide valuable information regarding future employment options, areas that need remediation and areas for which a future employer may need to make special accommodations (e.g., poor balance). In conjunction with the standardized test, job samples may also be presented. Tasks presented may include, but are not limited to 2-6 part assembly, sorting by size, shape, and color and packaging. Vocational interests are also determined through presentation of the Geist Picture Interest Inventory.

The evaluation results are combined with information from other sources (e.g., the resident record, resident living staff and activities therapy staff involved in the residents' programming) and a complete report is written concluding with recommendations. Test results may indicate that a work program is currently not appropriate as the resident has specific needs that preclude involvement (e.g., improvement in attention span). In such a case, alternate programming may be recommended. The evaluator may recommend a resident for a specific work placement based on several factors (such as test results, work interest, behavioral history, or staff ratio needs). Recommendations may be made regarding resident weaknesses displayed during testing and areas needing remediation (e.g., sensory ability or socialization). Recommendations to address other needs may be made, such as referral to the educational program to improve money-handling ability or to the behavioral program to reduce verbal aggression.

A variety of vocational training opportunities are provided on-grounds. The general purpose of these opportunities is to have clients work out of their residential unit and focus upon developing work habits and skills. Objectives for current clients focus on minimizing unnecessary verbal behavior, asking for more parts or materials as needed and reducing the number of prompts per session needed for the resident to continue working. Initial objectives may often focus upon the client staying at his/her assigned work station or not displaying aggressive behavior. In addition, work skill development is also a priority and clients are introduced to tasks which may be encountered in more advanced settings as well as actual tasks offered at the local work activity center.

Time studies are developed in order to provide working clients with a fair wage which is representative of their overall work quality and speed. Time studies have been formulated for housekeeping, woodworking, and production skills training placements provided on Oakdale Regional Center's campus. Times are averaged to determine an "industrial norm" which is the basis for the hourly wage to be assigned to the client following the time study. Findings are computed to obtain an hourly wage, and information is included in the client's record to indicate how his or her current hourly wage was obtained. Time studies are repeated at least every six months as required by law.

Clients who have demonstrated good work habits and skills are often referred for vocational training off campus. Some residents are employed in a community-based Prevocational Program/Work Activity Center at Growth and Opportunity, Inc., a local non-profit sheltered workshop. Depending upon the programs in which they are enrolled, they spend from 1/2 hour to 6 hours per day performing contracted production tasks such as steel-strap assembly or air vent assembly earning a piecework rate. Program emphasis may include developing task independence or improving work habits, such as staying on task and/or increasing production rates.

Other clients are employed in supported employment performing janitorial work provided through the Team Work, Inc., a local non-profit agency. Contracts include cleaning of banks, theaters and other job sites. Tasks include, but are not limited to, vacuuming, mopping, sweeping, picking up debris, and emptying trash containers. Program emphasis includes increasing compliance, working the entire session, and minimizing the number of verbal prompts to correctly complete assigned tasks.

Liaison

Coordination and communication between agencies is necessary in order to have an effective program which meets the client's need. An occupational therapist has been assigned to this task. The liaison is responsible for coordinating enrollment and for monitoring the clients in the program. Team meetings are convened to discuss client referrals and enrollment status and any problems that develop related to the program. Once a client is enrolled in the program, the liaison provides direct therapeutic services and/or consultations on a regular basis regarding program specifics. The liaison provides in-service training or sets up training sessions regarding adaptive equipment, positioning, passing medication and documentation guidelines. The liaison conducts annual occupational therapy evaluations, attends interdisciplinary team meetings, assists in the development of client's plan of service and serves as a consultant to resident units and referral agency.

As the major goal of all services provided within ORC is to prepare the resident for integration in community living, the team assessments and reviews will indicate appropriateness and readiness of the individual for referral to the Community Living Services division. This division of ORC services, in close coordination with the resident's interdisciplinary team, assumes responsibility for locating an appropriate community living setting and provides for a transition period including trial visits and new work settings or day programs as needed.

COMMUNITY LIVING SERVICES

The Community Living Services division of ORC operates under the same standards and regulations as the residential facility (ICF/MR and ACDD). The small group homes are ICF/MR certified, each independent and separate from that of the residential facility. The services provided by the division are predominately case management and professional consultation with direct client services provided by contract with various private practitioners, non-profit corporations and health care providers.

The development and management of all contracts, now totaling over $19.4 million per year along with the supervision of all the professional consultation services (medical, nursing, psychology and therapeutic services) is the responsibility of the Administrative-Clinical Support Services Director, a registered occupational therapist.

The Community Living Services division provides or arranges for occupational therapy evaluations and services to the approximately 440 residents served in the community. These individuals reside in approximately 80 different residential settings throughout the region. Groups of six or fewer individuals comprise these settings. The individuals range in age from 7 years to approximately 80 years. The placement and living arrangement is determined through the Interdisciplinary Team process which assures that all aspects of the individual's life are assessed prior to a specific placement.

All direct occupational therapy services are provided through a clinical services contractual relationship. The relationship may be with a private practitioner, a home health care agency, a community hospital, or with a county Community Mental Health Services Board. The provision of these services by individuals/agencies in the community where the individuals reside is one of the cornerstone philosophies of community placement. The individual in community placement receives as many services as possible from the same providers who provide services to the general population of the area.

The contract is a general document developed for all clinical support services with a specific attachment for occupational therapy services. The body of the document discusses the fact that financing is through Medicaid (Title XIX) and the responsibilities of the service provider, including confidentiality, maintaining insurance liability, civil rights issues and recipient rights. The Štandards, billing and charges for occupational therapy services cover such areas as:

1. direct provision of service through personal contact with the resident;
2. resident record documentation requirements and content areas to be included in evaluations;
3. statement of treatment plans in measurable goals and objectives;
4. participation requirements for interdisciplinary team meetings;
5. documentation of valid occupational therapy certification;
6. procedures for billings for services; and
7. authorized reimbursement rates.

The specific oversight of the occupational therapy, physical therapy, speech and recreational service contracts is provided by a Therapeutic Service Coordinator, a registered occupational therapist. The Coordinator assures that requests for services and billings are all in compliance with applicable standards and regulations.

The Therapeutic Services Coordinator assures that the contract occupational therapist utilizes the required annual evaluation format in completing the assessment, the same format as utilized at the Center (see Appendix 1). The contract therapist attends the interdisciplinary team meeting and as appropriate presents for discussion occupational therapy service programs for the individual, as well as recommendations for the overall needs of the individual.

When goals and objectives developed by the contractual therapist are to be delivered by the resident living staff of the home, the occupational therapist will provide inservice training to the staff on the rationale, implementation and documentation of the program. The therapist will then monitor and assure progress on a regularly scheduled basis. A schedule for training and observation is arranged, and the program is implemented as soon as possible after development and interdisciplinary team approval. Service areas include self-care, advanced daily living skills, prevocational skills, physical motor and cognitive/perceptual skills. The in-home programs are to be developed to complement the day program component of the service plan and vice versa. All progress is evaluated by a designated qualified mental retardation professional (QMRP) at least monthly.

The need for and appropriateness of adaptive assistive devices is assessed at least annually. The therapist may contact the Therapeutic Service Coordinator to acquire consultation from other professionals as necessary in determining the need for as well as the specific type of adaptive assistive device. When a device is chosen and obtained, the therapist provides inservice training to the individual and the resident living staff as to its care and use. The therapist will then follow up as necessary.

CONCLUSION

The utilization of occupational therapists within this regional services delivery system is extremely broad and diverse. It includes such positions as the agency director, specific program directors, the previously cited Administrative-Clinical Support Service Director and the Therapeutic Service Coordinator. Occupational therapists supervise the work training program and provide the liaison with community day program services. Contractual service occupational therapists serve the needs of residents in the small group homes throughout the service region.

We believe that the philosophical basis of the profession and the nature of occupational therapy education makes occupational therapists uniquely qualified for the diversity of roles and professional settings. Unfortunately the scarcity of qualified therapists results in the employment of fewer therapists than desired in many operations. Despite these shortages, more and more practicing therapists are finding increased opportunities to serve clients with developmental disabilities through their private practices and through contracts with community health care providers.

The goal for every resident within the ORC is that of community placement. All efforts of the facility staff are directed toward achieving that goal. To that extent, it has often been said that the mission of the facility is to put itself out of business. The decreasing resident population trends certainly reinforce that perspective. As the facility was reduced in size, the remaining populations steadily increased in percentages of persons with multiple and severely handicapping conditions since the lesser disabled persons were more easily assimilated into community programs. We have found, however, that degree of disability, severity of disorder or multiplicity of conditions are not deterrents to successful community living. The lack of coordinated planning, inaccessibility of services, community resistance to establishment of group homes, and our own lack of creativity are often the barriers that need to be overcome.

No doubt changes will continue to occur in the regional services system model. Occupational therapy plays a significant role in the delivery of services in today's implementation of that system. As these systems change and evolve the future role of occupational therapy will be what we as a profession and health care policymakers choose for the future. Our experience to date tells us that we must remain flexible and open to new ideas and concepts, prepared to assume leadership when opportunity allows and be professionally oriented to assure that all persons with developmental disabilities, regardless of their types of handicap, are provided with the highest possible level of services from appropriately trained professionals.

REFERENCES

The Accreditation Council on Services for People with Developmental Disabilities. (1987). *Standards for People with Developmental Disabilities*. Boston, MA.

Lederman, E.F. (1984). *Occupational Therapy in Mental Retardation*. Springfield, IL: Charles C. Thomas.

OAKDALE REGIONAL CENTER
Lapeer, Michigan 48446

(Name)

(Case Number)

PROGRAM Occupational Therapy

(Home)

ANNUAL EVALUATION

Birthdate: Age:

Evaluation Date:

Physician:

Referred by: (Name, Title)

Diagnosis:

Vision: Hearing:

Medications: (optional)

Precautions:

Equipment/Prothesis/Assistive Devices:

General Observations/Behavior:

Tests Administered:

Developmental/Reflexive level:

Physical Motor Skills: (include ROM, strength, coordination, grasp-release,
  sensation)

Activities of Daily Living:
    Self-Care: (include hygiene, dressing, feeding - include independence
               and oral-motor ability, balance, transfer, etc.)

    Community Living Skills: (include safety-judgment, household tasks,
                               clothes selection, time, money, etc.)

Cognitive-Perceptual-Motion: (include cognition, learning potential,
                               motivation, attention span, visual perception,
                               etc.)

Vocational-Prevocational: (include matching colors, size-shape discrimination)

Socialization: (include cooperative behavior, direction following mood, etc.)

Communication: (include how they communicate and ability to make themselves
                 understood)

Interests/Leisure Activities: (recreational, hobbies, etc. Should include
                               recreational likes/dislikes, what has been
                               done in past year and recommendations)

Clinical Impressions/Prognosis/Summary:

Current Programs:

Recommendations: 1) should be 2 types — a general and b-specific to
discipline; 2) prioritize; 3) give rationale

1.
2.
3.

_____
Signature - Title

On the Formative Stages
of the Adult Screening Questionnaire:
A Managerial Approach for Screening
Adult Developmentally Disabled Clients

Sharon Lefkofsky, MS, OTR
Tamara E. Avi-Itzhak, DSc

SUMMARY. This article describes the formative stages of a screening tool for developmentally disabled adults, the Adult Screening Questionnaire (ASQ). ASQ offers occupational therapists a uniform approach for screening clients. Employing the ASQ will result with a client profile that leads to improved capability in screening outcomes for service delivery: prioritizing caseloads, identifying domains of need for comprehensive evaluation, facilitating clinical decision making, and reporting population needs to administrators. These screening outcomes contribute to determining the client eval-

Sharon Lefkofsky has worked in developmental disabilities for thirty years as an educator, program developer, and clinician. She has been on the innovative edge of program development in developmental disabilities in Michigan and in New York in both policy and practice issues. She has been with New York University as Program Coordinator for the post professional degree program with specialization in developmental disabilities for the past seven years. Previously, she was on faculty at Wayne State University in Detroit, Michigan. Presently, she is a doctoral candidate at New York University. Tamara E. Avi-Itzhak is currently Adjunct Associate Professor at New York University, Department of Occupational Therapy, and Clinical Associate Professor at City University of New York (CUNY), Health Science Center at Brooklyn, New York, teaching research courses to graduate students. Previously, she was a faculty member at the University of Haifa, Israel, for the Schools of Education and Occupational Therapy. She was editor of the *Journal for Studies in Organization and Educational Administration*. She was Director of Center for Education Administration at University of Haifa.

107

uation and program intervention necessary for the service delivery process.

Reported are rationale for the development/use of the instrument, previous validity studies, modifications, and pilot study testing for reliability. The Clients Profile will enable the clinicians to establish three priority levels according to clients' needs. In addition, each client's needs are identified on nine domains of occupational therapy programmatic concern. A summary of findings for five outcomes for service delivery is introduced. Limitations and plans for further modification and study are discussed.

INTRODUCTION

This article describes the formative stages of the development of the Adult Screening Questionnaire (ASQ). The ASQ makes it possible for occupational therapists to employ a uniform approach for screening a new group of adult developmentally delayed adults. Employing this screening tool will result in a client profile that leads the individual therapist to improved capability in the following screening outcomes for service delivery: (a) prioritize caseloads, (b) identify domain/s of need for occupational therapy service, (c) assist in determining further areas for assessment, (d) facilitate clinical decision making, and (e) report population needs to administrators. These screening outcomes along with client evaluation, program intervention, and program evaluation constitute the service delivery process. These screening outcomes contribute to determining the client evaluation and program intervention neces-

The mailing address for both authors: New York University, Department of Occupational Therapy, 34 Stuyvesant St., New York, NY 10003.

The authors would like to acknowledge the following people. Charlotte Exner, MA, OTR, Towsen University for sharing results of her research of the original Adult Screening Questionnaire, and encouraging the further testing of the tool. Michael Chapman, Director, The Kennedy Institute, Department for Community Services, Baltimore, Maryland for written permission to modify the ASQ for occupational therapists for use in both community and institutional settings. Dalia Sachs, PhD, Haifa University and N.Y.U., for computer analyses. Lise Hershkowitz, MS, OTR, Neal Harvison, OTR, work/study students at N.Y.U., and Tzwe Shin Howe, MS, OTR, and Larry Zachow, MS, OTR, doctoral candidates at N.Y.U., all employed by OMRDD of New York State, for assistance with revisions, data collection, and testing.

sary for the service delivery process (Halpern et al., 1982; Halpern, 1986).

Since developmentally delayed individuals present a complex set of problems and services to these individuals are not unlimited, identifying such a tool is essential. Even an experienced occupational therapist can feel overwhelmed when confronted with the difficulties of prioritizing a caseload from the total existing population. In addition to establishing a priority caseload, the therapist must make a clinical decision with regards to which domain occupational therapy intervention should be focused upon for a given client.

The above concerns, plus the need for a uniform approach to screening, led to the search for an existing screening tool that would give focus to the occupational therapist in the management of his/ her caseload. The rationale for the choice of the ASQ was based on convincing validity tests performed by its originators.

The ASQ was developed by Charlotte Exner for the Kennedy Institute, Department for Community Services, Baltimore, Maryland. The Kennedy Institute granted written permission for the first author to modify the ASQ in 1986. Further elaboration will follow later in this paper.

The article includes a section on background information which provides rationale for the development/use of the instrument. Previous validity studies, modifications made by the authors, and pilot study testing for reliability are reported. *Clients Profile*, the summary of findings, demonstrates the ASQ's capacity for improving the five outcomes for service delivery mentioned above and will be introduced. Finally, limitations and plans for further modification and study are discussed.

BACKGROUND AND NEED

Measurement of Outcome in Developmental Disabilities

In his chapter, Halpern (1986), has offered an analysis of the issues of measurement in mental retardation and use of uniform terminology along with a decision-making model for the service delivery process. This analysis and the decision-making model reflect shifts which have occurred in the past two decades from emphasis on classification and diagnosis of mentally retarded to the assessment of the service delivery process.

Measurement of Outcome in the Context of Service Delivery

Traditional measurement of persons with mental retardation (hereinafter referred to as M.R.) were mainly psychometric ones and were driven by the concept and definition of mental retardation. Due to the psychometric nature of these measures, they concentrated on incidence, prevalence, and prevention. In addition, the assessments were often not originated for the specific needs of persons with M. R. Furthermore, these assessments were often administered in isolated settings removed from the environment where the behavior usually occurs. Such assessments did not have characteristics for testing skill attainment and community adjustment.

Another related issue of measurement is format. The two basic formats which appear representative of contemporary assessment of persons with retardation are tests and rating scales (Halpern et al., 1982, p.9-99). While tests require some behavior on the part of the person being tested, rating scales involve judgement of a reporter, a third person, who describes the behavior of the client being evaluated. Each format has strengths and weaknesses: the rating scale is criticized as being more susceptible to errors of judgement. The rating scale is generally considered a better estimate of performance over time. Tests permit a limited number of opportunities to respond to test items. The advantage is that one has the opportunity to view actual performance. The chosen format for the ASQ is the rating scale. This decision was based on time restraints, client availability, and performance variances.

These traditional measurement practices did not contribute to the service delivery process as presently perceived. Furthermore, these measurements posed methodological problems related to their validity and reliability.

The most current definition of mental retardation issued in 1983 by the American Association of Mental Retardation (Grossman, 1983) essentially has three components which contribute to the service delivery process. These are intelligence, developmental period, and adaptive behavior. Intelligence serves only for the purpose of documenting an impairment whereas raising the intelligence is not considered as a goal of the habilitation process (Halpern, 1986, p.30). Developmental period is generally interpreted to mean the initial diagnosis which occurred before the age of eighteen. Adaptive behavior, replacing the traditional term of social competence, serves as an indicator for the repertoire of social skills. This term was changed because of the ambiguity of the concept of social competence.

Essentially, people with mental retardation are viewed as having a limited repertoire of social skills and limited insight into the causes and consequences of their behavior. This concept is inherent in all definitions of mental retardation (Halpern, 1986, 1982).

Adaptive behavior is frequently included in the goals of habilitation as an attempt to reduce disability (i.e., improving skills), or as an attempt to reduce the handicap (i.e., providing opportunities to enjoy socially valued roles) (Brolin, 1983; Halpern, 1986; Wolfsenberger, 1972). Adaptive behavior is an integral component of the definition of mental retardation and an appropriate target for outcome assessment.

The service delivery process suggested by Halpern (1982), corresponds with the current perception of the service delivery process in that the process assesses ability to perform functional tasks in a variety of environments. In essence, Halpern's model includes four stages of decision making: needs assessment, program planning, program implementation and monitoring, and program evaluation. A strength of the model is the proposed linkage, through assessment information, of decisions made during each step of the service delivery process. When such linkage occurs, it provides support for the accountability requirements of continued service delivery. It is of interest to note that this service delivery process is parallel to the occupational therapy process (Hopkins and Tiffany, 1983; Day, 1973).

ASQ is a needs assessment activity which is part of the first component of Halpern's (1982) model in the sense that it leads to decisions which affect both eligibility determination and setting of service priorities. Eligibility in the context of the ASQ refers to the priority setting goal stated earlier. In other words, eligibility determines those needing occupational therapy services rather than eligibility in the broader sense of generalized service delivery. We regard the function of the ASQ as similar in nature and parallel to the Parachek Geriatric Rating Scale (Parachek and King, 1976; Fidler, 1984), which serves to determine eligibility for psychiatric and geriatric clients. Eligibility is the function of interface between individual needs and environmental opportunities (Halpern, 1982; Fidler, 1984, pp.45-50). Fidler (1984) stresses the importance of early needs assessment of patients admitted to formulate a treatment plan and to set priorities. Under her model, needs assessment activity includes goal determination for each discipline as well as identification of client needs. This combination of activity addresses the importance of the interface between individual needs and environmental opportunity. Fidler's concept of needs assessment and the concrete example of the Parachek served as an impetus to the development of the ASQ.

Level of Retardation

Two interpretations for dealing with the level of retardation are suggested in the literature. Fuhrer (1986, pp.146-7) suggests using descriptions of general levels of function that are on a continuum and which include: independent—complete independence or modified independence; dependent—modified dependence or complete dependence. Halpern (1982) on the other hand, suggests that subtests within a given assessment should be identified as appropriate for each level of retardation: mildly, moderately, severely, or severely or profoundly retarded.

The ASQ in its current edition subsumes Fuhrer and Halpern's interpretations with respect to levels of retardation. The ASQ's revised edition is comprised of specific items relevant to both poles of the continuum of the levels of retardation. This modification was made to accommodate the tool to multiple environments (community residence, day care center, or institution), so that occupational therapists can extend the screening process to include a broader range in the continuum of the level of mental retardation as well as the continuum of function. Therefore, occupational therapists using the ASQ can evaluate both higher and lower levels of retardation as well as evaluating higher and lower levels of function. The ASQ is capable of depicting all possible combinations of different levels of retardation with levels of function.

Uniform Terminology System

The Functional Independent Measure (FIM) developed in 1983, is a uniform national data system for medical rehabilitation. The system was developed by recommendation to Congress for a patient classification system, coding system, and uniform patient assessment instrument so that rehabilitation "products" could be defined accurately (Hamilton in Fuhrer, 1986, p.138). The result was a system that would document the outcomes of medical rehabilitation.

The American Occupational Therapy Association (AOTA) was a sponsor of the Task Force for FIM. This sponsorship resulted in the development of three outcome products. These outcome products were completed in 1985 and are the following: (1) a Uniform System for Reporting Occupational Therapy Services, (2) a proposed Occupational Therapy Product Output Reporting System, and (3) a Uniform Occupational Therapy Evaluation Checklist (Bair & Gwin, 1985, pp.5-16). It is the expectation that eventually all practicing occupational therapists will be using the uniform data system.

The two systems for uniform terminology interface because the conceptual foundation is similar in that it characterizes and defines the rehabilitation process. The rehabilitation process serves as the basis for the development of the uniform data system. It follows that many categories are also similar. The FIM and Uniform Terminology of AOTA selected a minimum number of key activities intended to be valid (necessary and sufficient) indicators of level of disability or cost of disability.

The ASQ includes uniform terminology language as well as certain categories of the Uniform Terminology System.

Occupational Therapy Content and the ASQ

Use of Reed's model of adaptation through occupation (Reed, 1984) fits with AAMD's conceptual definition of mental retardation, which reflects the uniqueness of occupational therapy. Under Reed's model, occupational therapy is concerned with the activities or routines of daily living within a given time and space and the meaning of those activities in terms of adaptive behavior for that individual. According to Reed (1984), "adaptation through occupation means the organization and management of occupational activities and tasks in a manner that meets the goal of achieving maximum autonomy or functional independence, actualization or satisfaction and accomplishment" (p.495). Many professions have similar goals for the client.

The key to the uniqueness of occupational therapy intervention is through occupation. Under the occupational therapy model, occupation related activities are used to help people develop, restore or maintain a normal routine of occupational activities in self maintenance, productivity and leisure. Furthermore, by occupation Reed means those activities and tasks which a person performs as part of the daily living routine. These tasks should engage the individual's resources, time and energy (p.495).

Using Reed's model and two taxonomies of occupation and performance (p.494-6) helps to explain the conceptualization and delineation of the categories and the items chosen for inclusion in the Adult Screening Questionnaire.

Summary

The foregoing analysis provides the rationale for the development of a screening tool using outcome measures as a means of clinical decision making for service delivery by occupational therapists. A functional assessment is a profile of strengths and weaknesses along one or more dimensions of behavior relevant to a variety of environmental settings. Ultimately, the goal of a functional assessment is to identify problems which need professional intervention to help developmentally delayed clients reach higher levels of socially acceptable behavior, or adaptive behavior.

After weighing the methodological advantages and disadvantages of the rating scale format, the authors decided to retain this format. This decision was based on the results of analysis of the pilot study and discussion conducted with individual therapists involved with the pilot. In addition, the use of uniform terminology in the ASQ results in a uniform data system that can be applied to assessment. The content model for occupational therapy presents a compatible conceptualization with contemporary assessment methodology and management of service provision.

THE INSTRUMENT AND INSTRUMENTATION

ASQ is a prescreening tool designed to assist occupational therapists in identifying adolescents and adults with developmental disabilities who are in need of comprehensive occupational therapy evaluations. The tool is comprised of individual items designed to address nine content domains of occupational therapy:

    1-4: ADL Skills(oral-motor/eating, dressing, hygiene, and homemaking)
    5: Community and ADL
    6: Job Tasks, Leisure Activities and ADL
    7: Motor Aspects
    8: Sensory, Perceptual, Cognitive Aspects
    9: Social, Emotional Aspects

Development and Previous Research

The ASQ was originally developed by The Kennedy Institute,* Baltimore, Maryland, in response to inappropriate referrals that had been made for occupational therapy and physical therapy services for developmentally disabled adults in community residences (Interview, Exner 1986,7). The Kennedy Institute generated the development of the ASQ, and a clinical researcher interviewed administrators, adult care staff, and clients to survey their perceptions and understanding of occupational and physical therapy services. The outcome of The Kennedy Institute's study resulted in Adult Screening Questionnaires in Occupational Therapy and Physical Therapy as well as in Communications, Nutrition, and Wheelchair Positioning and Use.

The results of studies testing face and sampling validity of the ASQ showed that the tool was free of jargon and that the content was appropriate and adequate. These results were derived from pro-

---

*The Adult Screening Questionnaire was developed by Charlotte Exner for The Kennedy Institute, Department for Community Services, Baltimore, Maryland. The Kennedy Institute, granted written permission for the author to modify the Adult Screening Questionnaire in 1986. The choice to use and modify an existing tool rather than create a new one, was made on advice from consultants. Additional validation studies by Kennedy Institute on the Adult Screening Tool had already been done and were considered important.

cedures involving occupational therapists interviewing supervisors of/and direct care staff in the first stage. In the second stage, an occupational therapist external to Kennedy Institute reviewed completed interviews to determine the need for comprehensive evaluation. Results indicate a 93% agreement of need of comprehensive evaluation between outside reviewers and inside staff.

Furthermore, additional results indicate the existence of a match between individual items within the domains under assessment as well as items within each of those domains.

Administration and Instrumentation

To administer the questionnaire, an interview is conducted by the occupational therapist with a third party (either a direct care staff or a supervisor of a program for a developmentally disabled individual). Following a debriefing period, the purpose of the questionnaire is stated and the instructions for answering the questions are reviewed. During the 15-20 minute (approximate) time period, responses are recorded by placing a checkmark in one of the following three ranked columns titled, "yes"(l), "sometimes"(2), or "no"(3). The instruction sheet directs the interviewee to answer "yes" if: (a) the answer is yes or true, or (b) the person consistently completes the skill without physical or verbal assistance from others, and (c) the person consistently completes the skill within a reasonable amount of time. The answer to the question should be "sometimes" if (a) the person is inconsistent doing the skill independently, or (b) occasionally demonstrates the ability , or (c) occasionally needs additional time. The answer to the question should be "no" if, (a) the answer is no or false, or (b) the person is unable to complete the skill, or (c) the person never completes the skill without additional physical or verbal assistance from others, or (d) the person is unable to complete the skill in a reasonable amount of time.

The scoring is done by the occupational therapist. Each client receives nine summed scores on items comprising each of the above listed domains. These scores serve as individual indicators of need for occupational therapy intervention in each of the specific areas of domain.

The tool offers a quick, systematic analysis of client needs. The scoring of the questionnaire and its subsections will provide the therapist with the information to design and implement a comprehensive model of service delivery, which is cost and time effective.

Modifications/Field Testing

Revisions and modifications to the original tool were performed in order to achieve the following objectives: (1) the questionnaire will be used in institutional as well as community settings; (2) the interview method will replace a self reporting questionnaire; and (3) the tool will be cost effective and parsimonious. The three stages of modification executed reflect the above mentioned objectives.

Thus, the first stage represents the first field test of the ASQ in that it was administered in an institution (see Table 1). Not only was the environment changed but also the administration methodology. Clients were evaluated by direct observation in conjunction with the ASQ; the ASQ was also self administered; and, the ASQ was administered by the interview method. Based on these attempts, results indicated that the ASQ was a viable tool in the institutional setting as well as the community setting. These were encouraging results as occupational therapists practice in both settings. Furthermore, the results of the first stage indicated that the interview was far more suitable in the institutions under investigation.

In the second stage, items were added to the ASQ to include special needs of lower functioning clients. These items were subjected to additional tests for language clarity and validity. While the first two stages represent attempts to accommodate for environmental and methodological aspects, the third stage was performed in order to achieve cost effectiveness. The number of items was reduced from 64 items to 49 items. This was accomplished by reliability tests which will be discussed in the next section.

As indicated earlier, these modifications reflect results from field tests and incorporated feedback from clinicians, direct care staff and their supervisors. Some items were not applicable and others were redundant. Those items which were appropriate for the higher functioning client were left on the ASQ to accommodate a variety of mentally retarded with different levels of function.

TABLE 1. Summary of Modifications of the ASQ: Domain

Domain	First Stage		Second Stage		Third Stage	
	# of Items	Maximum	# of Items	Maximum	# of Items	Maximum
I Oral-Motor/ Eating Skills	11	33	12	36	8	24
II Dressing	4	12	4	12	3	9
III Hygiene	9	27	10	30	6	18
IV Homemaking	6	18	6	18	6	18
V Community And Other ADL Skills	5	15	5	15	4	12
VI Job Tasks, ADL, And Leisure Activities	2	6	2	6	2	6
VII Motor Aspects	9	27	9	27	7	21
VIII Sensory/Perceptual/ Cognitive Aspects	10	30	11	33	10	30
IX Social/Emotional Aspects	6	18	5	15	3	9
TOTAL	62	186	64	192	49	147

The third modification was made to reduce the items found to be redundant in the first and second revisions. In the following section, the specific reliability tests that were performed in order to achieve the aforementioned objectives will be illustrated. See Table 1 for summary of the three stages.

RELIABILITY TESTS

Interrater Reliability Pilot Test

An interrater reliability (function of agreement) test was performed on the first stage of the ASQ on 12 subjects. The test was done according to the formula suggested by Polit and Hungler (1983, p.391). Results of this test appear on Table 2 and indicate that a high degree of interrater reliability exists, r = .93.

Internal Consistency Reliability Test

This reliability test was performed on the second stage of the revision. The sample consisted of interviews of 70 direct care staff reporting on their clients. The clients are adults who are severely-profoundly mentally retarded and multiply handicapped. The clients live in "apartment-like" units contained within a remodeled institutional building considered to be a transition home from the

TABLE 2. Equivalence (Interobserver) Reliability (Function of Agreements): Pilot Test (N = 12)

Elements	Formula	Coefficient of Agreement
	$r = \dfrac{N}{N + K} =$	
where:		
N = Number of Agreements	$\dfrac{61}{61 + 4}$	= .93
K = Number of Disagreements		

institution to the community. The clients attend a day program in the building in which they live. The direct care staff are assigned to clients for feeding, dressing, and goal directed programs.

The interview was conducted in a quiet room away from the distractions of the dayroom, which is the center of activity. The interviewer, an occupational therapist, read the instructions to the interviewee, proceeding with the questionnaire, and clarifying when necessary. The interviews lasted approximately 15 minutes, and the scoring was done by the therapist. Demographic and medical variables, including age, type of program, diagnosis, medications, and associated problems, were obtained from the individual client record at another time.

One of the most widely used methods for internal consistency testing, namely, Cronbach's alpha, was employed (Chronbach, 1978). Results of the test performed on one of the nine domains (chosen at random) comprising the instrument, Sensory/Perception/Cognition Aspects, appear on Table 3. Data show that the reliability coefficient (Cronbach's alpha) equaling .68 is regarded as an acceptable level of reliability (Nunnally, 1978).

In essence, the coefficient obtained shows that these ten items are indeed measuring the same domain: Sensory /Perceptual/Cognitive Aspects. Furthermore, results suggest that by eliminating items 1, 2, or 3, we may somewhat improve the value of the coefficient and at the same time achieve a tool with a higher parsimony. Future decisions about item configuration will be made following additional testing of the fourth modified version which is in process.

Stability Test

The stability test of reliability was performed on the same data obtained for the internal consistency reliability test. The results of this test are presented on Table 4.

Results of the Pearson correlation coefficients performed on items which are obviously related (chosen at random) range from $r = .17$; $p = .05$ for "lose liquid from mouth when eating" and "drink from a glass," to $r = .75$; $p = .001$ for "lose liquid from mouth when eating" and "lose liquid from mouth when drinking."

The values of these coefficients, and in fact, all other coefficients enable us to suggest that the ASQ in its present revision exhibits satisfactory levels of reliability. These results are encouraging and indicate the relative merits of the tool.

Clients' Profiles

Table 5 represents findings pertaining to three of the nine domains (chosen at random) included in the ASQ. These findings represent clients' profiles in that they summarize needs in quantifiable measures which are not only absolute but also relative in nature. They are absolute in the sense that the measure represents each individual's need as a client. They are relative in the sense that the measure represents the needs of the total group for occupational therapy evaluation in any one of the three domains. Thus, an overall profile would be one which includes the scores of all the nine domains.

To illustrate the process of developing a profile of clients, turn to Table 5, #3, the Motor Aspects domain. This table presents a distribution of scores on Motor Aspects domain by need for evaluation. There are nine items measuring these skills in the ASQ. The minimum score a client can receive in this domain is nine. Thus, clients not needing any further evaluation in this domain would receive a score of nine and will be regarded as third priority for evaluation. The clients most in need of evaluation will receive a score of 27 and will be regarded as most in need of further evaluation.

The range of the actual scores in this domain of the sample under investigation for this particular domain (N = 70) was 9-25. Once the actual range was established, it was divided into three levels of priority of need. The first priority, those who scored between 15-25 are most in need of evaluation. Data show that there are 29 (42%) such clients. The second level of priority includes those somewhat in need. There are 26 (37%) clients in this group. There are 15 (21%) clients in the third priority level who scored 9. Those clients are not in need of occupational therapy evaluation.

Clients' profiles will enable the occupational therapist to communicate to the administration concrete data about the need for services of the entire group as well as identify groups of clients in need of evaluation within the individual domains. As for the individual

TABLE 3. Internal Consistency Reliability: (Cronbach's Alpha) Total Population (N = 70)

Domain	Individual Items	Alpha if item deleted

Sensory/Perceptual/Cognitive

1. Have (or appear to have) a usual problem that affects use of materials and tools? .70

2. Become upset with normal touch from other people and/or objects? .70

3. Seem afraid of simple movement activities that are within their physical ability (going up/down stairs, climbing on a small ladder, etc.)? .72

4. Seem to be unaware of body parts or body size--often bumps into objects or people, falls when attempting to sit down in a chair, etc.? .68

5. Seem to ignore one side of the body; and/or seem to 'forget' that one hand exists? .68

6. Seem to have difficulty in learning the sequence of steps involved in completing a task? .65

7. Have a good attention span—stay on task despite normal distractions in the environment? .63

8. Match and sort objects according to color, shape and/or size? .62

9. Remember how to do tasks or skills after they are presented several times? .60

10. Remember the sequence of activities to be performed during a typical day and where to go/where to do these activities? .59

N = 70   N of items = 10   Reliability Coefficient = .68
Cronbach's Alpha

TABLE 4. Stability Test (obviously related items): Pearson Correlation, Total Population (N = 70)

Item		1.	2.	
	Oral Motor Skills			
1.	Loose liquid from mouth when eating?	--		
2.	Loose liquid from mouth when drinking?	.75***	--	

Item		3.	4.	5.
	Eating Skills			
3.	Eat appropriate foods with their fingers?	--		
4.	Eat with a spoon?	.68**	--	
5.	Drink from a glass?	.69**	.45**	--

ITEM		1.	2.
1.	Loose liquid from mouth when eating?	--	
2.	Drink from a glass?	.17*	--

*** p = .001
 ** p = .01
  * p = .05

therapist, these profiles promote efficient program planning for resources allocation of both manpower and equipment. Additionally, the profile can assist in determining the model(s) for intervention according to the clients needs and the nature of the setting.

Being able to arrive at a quantifiable measure for clients' needs provides evidence for the accountability requirements of continued service delivery whose relevance cannot be stressed enough. This provision goes hand in hand with Christiansen's (1983) warning

TABLE 5. Need Assessment: Clients Profiles Total Population (N = 70)

Domain	Number of Items	Theoretical Range	Actual Range	1st Priority N (%)	2nd Priority N (%)	3rd Priority N (%)
1. Oral/Motor/Eating skills*	11	11-33	11-31	17-31 22 (47%)	12-16 21 (47%)	11 3 (6%)
2. Sensory/Perceptual/Cognitive Aspects	10	10-30	10-27	16-27 34 (50%)	11-15 28 (40%)	10 7 (10%)
3. Motor Aspects	9	9-27	9-25	15-25 29 (42%)	10-14 26 (37%)	9 15 (21%)

*N=46 (where knife is offered)

that those professions which can demonstrate accountability by quantifiable means will be the professions which will survive.

Limitations and Recommendations

Introducing a screening tool is not an easy task and should be regarded as an ongoing process. It should be mentioned that a characteristic of the early reliability effort was based on random selection of domain as well as items within a domain because we wanted some degree of assurance of the ASQ's reliability before comprehensive efforts of systems testing was made.

One issue that needs to be addressed is the further reduction of items for improved cost effectiveness. In addition, some test items were found to be too wordy and ambiguous; indeed, the original authors may have added additional statements for clarification. These statements are superfluous in the newer format. Further reductions in items and within the items cannot be achieved without further testing and retesting of the ASQ, and, at the present time, additional testing is underway for both reliability and validity.

Another issue that needs to be further addressed is the fact that there is no discrimination built in the ASQ to differentiate between not being able to function and not being allowed to function. For example, if a client is not offered a fork or a knife, there is no way to determine if the client has the ability to perform this function or is denied the opportunity to perform this function.

A surprising response to the screening process was that of the occupational therapists participating in the early revisions. These occupational therapists said they were uncomfortable with the screening process. This response, in part, could be because occupational therapists are traditionally trained to do in-depth evaluations rather than use a screening process. Secondly, they expressed discomfort using a third party for information gathering rather than using their own skills, especially when they perceive a discrepancy in the data given by the interviewee. This difficulty was anticipated when administrative options were explored, and a decision was made to use this format over other formats for reasons mentioned earlier.

The strength of the tool for the occupational therapist and for the person being interviewed is that the interview helps in establishing rapport, as demonstrated by the following comment from a field tester. For example, it was reported that the interview process was considered valuable by the person being interviewed, who stated, "my opinion is valued and someone really cares what I think."

We regard the Clients' Profile as a major outcome of the ASQ. We suggest that the levels of priority for evaluation should be regarded as flexible ones and should be based on actual ranges obtained for each individual domain. The priorities presented in Table 5 should serve as an empirical example. We recommend that the individual therapists not apply rigid rules for establishing the three ranges. One should be aware of the fact that the clients in the middle of the range are most vulnerable for being eliminated from further evaluation. Therefore, each domain should be considered independently.

CONCLUSION

As indicated earlier the ASQ has the potential and merits to fill in a gap in the service delivery process. It is of utmost importance to be able to incorporate empirical data as a source for comprehensive evaluation. As an efficient screening tool, the ASQ facilitates appropriate service delivery to adults with mental retardation thereby bringing involvement in community life one step closer (Taylor, 1988).

In addition, the ASQ also facilitates the clinician in responding to professional and administrative needs. This tool quantifies work loads based on the needs of the clients. This in turn leads to guidelines for implementation of appropriate service to those in need. As specific treatment plans are established, professional manpower needs can be identified for future hiring. The quantifying of work loads is another advantage for clinicians who need to account for their time in the competitive health care system.

The main advantages of ASQ could be summarized as follows: (a) prioritize caseloads, (b) identify domain/s of need for occupational therapy service, (c) assist in determining further areas of assessment, (d) facilitate clinical decision making, and (e) report population needs to administrators.

REFERENCES

Bair, J. & Gwin, C. (Eds.). (1985). *A productivity systems guide for occupational therapy*. Maryland: American Occupational Therapy Association, Inc.

Brolin, J. (1983). *Life centered career education* (2nd rev. ed.). Virginia: Council for Exceptional Children.

Christiansen, C. H. (1983). Research: An economic imperative [editorial]. *Occupational Therapy Journal of Research*, Vol. 3, No. 4, pp. 195-198.

Cronbach, L. J. (1970). *Essentials of psychological testing* (3rd ed.). New York: Harper and Row.

Day, D. A. (1973). System diagramming for teaching treatment planning. *American Journal of Occupational Therapy*, Vol. 27, No. 5, pp. 239-243.

Fidler, G. S. (1984). *Design of rehabilitation services in psychiatric hospital settings*. Maryland: Ramsco Publishing Company.

Fuhrer, M. J. (1986). *Rehabilitation outcomes: Analysis and measurement*. Baltimore: Paul Brookes.

Grossman, H. J. (1983). *Classification in mental retardation*. Washington, D.C.: American Association on Mental Deficiency.

Halpern, A. S. (1986). Outcome analysis for persons with mental retardation. In M. J. Fuhrer (Ed.), *Rehabilitation outcomes* (1984). Baltimore: Paul Brookes.

Halpern, A., Lehmann, J. P., Irvin, L. K., Heiry, & T. J. (1982). *Contemporary assessment for mentally retarded adolescents and adults*. Baltimore: University Park Press.

Hopkins, H. L. & Tiffany, E. G. (1983). Occupational therapy — a problem solving process. In H. L. Hopkins and M. D. Smith (Eds.), *Willard and Spackman's occupational therapy* (6th ed.). Philadelphia: Lippincott Company.

Nachmias, D. & Nachmias, C. (1987). *Research methods in the social sciences* (3rd ed.). New York: St. Martin's Press.

Nunnally, J. (1978). *Psychometric theory*. New York: McGraw-Hill.

Parachek, J. & King, L. J. (1976). *Parachek geriatric rating scale and treatment manuals*. Arizona: Greenroom Publications.

Polit, D. & Hungler, B. (1983). *Nursing research: Principles and methods* (2nd ed.). Philadelphia: Lippincott.

Reed, K. L. (1984). *Models of practice in occupational therapy*. Baltimore: Williams and Wilkins.

Taylor, S. J. (1988). Caught in the continuum: A critical analysis of the principle of the least restrictive environment. *Journal Association of Severely Handicapped*, Vol. 13, No. 1, pp. 41-53.

Thorndike, R. L. & Hagen, E. (1977). *Measurement and evaluation in psychology and education*. New York: J. Wiley and Sons.

Wolfensberger, W. (1972). *The principle of normalization in human services*. Toronto: National Institute on Mental Retardation.

Intervention Strategies for Promoting Feeding Skills in Infants with Sensory Deficits

Jane Case-Smith, EdD, OTR

SUMMARY. Feeding is multi-sensory, highly stimulating experience for infants and young children. Feeding interactions with children who have oral sensory processing deficits may be therapeutic and pleasurable or may be stressful and disorganizing. Specific oral motor and feeding problems in hyposensitive/hypotonic children and hypersensitive/hypertonic children are described. Occupational therapy intervention that emphasizes sensory stimulation related to the environment, handling before and during feeding, and the sensory qualities of food is explained.

INTRODUCTION

Occupational therapists work with infants to enhance and develop oral motor skills in feeding. Often therapy occurs during the feeding process. The feeding interaction between a mother or a therapist and an infant is a multi-sensory experience. This interaction combines tactile, gustatory, auditory, vision, and often vestibular stimulation. For the child with sensory processing deficits, the multi-sensory stimulation that occurs during feeding can be therapeutically arousing or uncomfortable and stressful. A basic knowledge of the normal oral sensory mechanisms and of oral sensory dysfunction is important to understand the therapeutic potentials and hazards of oral stimulation and feeding.

Jane Case-Smith is Assistant Professor at Virginia Commonwealth University. Her mailing address is 14771 Conway Drive, Manassas, VA 22111. This manuscript is based on a presentation at the 1988 AOTA Conference.

129

This paper describes the sensory mechanisms in and around the mouth. Oral motor development typical of children with hypo- or hyper-sensitivities is described, including an explanation of the feeding problems associated with oral sensory dysfunction. The concluding section discusses intervention strategies for infants and young children with oral sensory deficits. These strategies use therapeutic sensory stimulation to enhance oral motor skills and to promote positive feeding interactions.

ORAL SENSORY MECHANISMS

The lips and tongue have an abundance of sensory receptors. They are probably the most sensitive areas of the body, with up to 10 times more sensory receptors than other parts of the body. The lips are prehenders that perform intricate sequential movements and have more tactile receptors than our fingers (Thach, 1973). The tongue is similarly full of tactile receptors and also has the specialized taste receptors.

The oral sensory system develops intrauterine. The fetus first responds to touch in the perioral area at 7 1/2 fetal weeks. By 11 weeks swallowing movements occur when the lips are touched. By 29 weeks touch to the lips causes sucking movements (Rose, 1973). Primitive taste is present in the 30 week old preemie. Full term newborns can differentiate between good nutrient taste and foul taste (Nowlis, 1973). In conclusion, the oral structures have an abundance of sensory receptors that are functional very early in life.

The jaw, tongue, and lips are well supplied with muscle spindles that relay proprioceptive information to motor neurons and are directly responsible for reflexive jaw, tongue, and lip movement. Because the tongue and jaw muscles have well developed proprioceptive mechanisms, many of the oral movements operate through the muscle spindle reflex arc rather than through higher level cortical control (Kawamura & Morimotor, 1973). During feeding, tongue, lips, and cheeks respond automatically to the sensory qualities of food. Oral afferents travel via the facial and glossopharyngeal nerves to the lower brainstem nuclei. Some of these afferents synapse directly onto the trigeminal and hypoglossal motor nuclei (Kawamura & Morimotor, 1973). Therefore, oral sensory input produces a direct, automatic motor response from these brainstem nuclei.

The trigeminal nerve carries proprioceptive messages from the tongue and jaw and relays a return motor signal of reciprocal strength to the tongue and jaw muscles. The trigeminal nerve has other tracks which reach higher brain centers, carrying messages of diffuse touch, pain, temperature, pressure, and proprioception from the oral area (Chusid, 1976). Tracks of this nerve lead to the thalamus and to the cerebellum. Projections from the thalamus travel to the parietal lobe. A number of axonal projections terminate in the reticular formation where the information is joined by messages from other sensory systems.

The multitude of connections from the oral area to the reticular activating center explains why oral tactile stimulation is highly arousing and alerting. Farber (1982) and Rood (1962) both emphasize touch to the oral area for achieving general inhibition or excitation of the nervous system. Farber advocates use of deep pressure on the lips for total inhibition of body movement and light brushing for alerting and arousal.

Both gustatory and olfactory systems have connections to the limbic system (Farber, 1982). Therefore, the sensory input that occurs during feeding travels to the system which mediates our emotions. In addition, individuals receive and express affection through touch to the lips, and these tactile receptors in the lips and oral structures also send messages to the limbic system. The lips are known to be erotic areas and the intensity of general arousal and stimulation of emotional response should not be underestimated.

Touch and taste are only two of the sensory systems stimulated during feeding. Visual, auditory, and vestibular systems may simultaneously be stimulated. Tracks of these sensory systems converge on the reticular activating system, affecting arousal level (Farber, 1982). The sensory experience of feeding seems to have multiple effects on the child. Feeding may create a strong emotional response. Typically, feeding is a wonderful, even erotic sensory experience, and children derive great pleasure from the taste and texture of food as well as the other sensory stimuli which often accompany the feeding experience. Therapists need to realize the intensity of feeding as a sensory experience which should result in pleasure to the child and reciprocally enjoyment for the parent.

FEEDING PROBLEMS IN CHILDREN
WITH SENSORY DEFICITS

Oral sensory problems may be exemplified by two types of children, those who are hyposensitive and those who are hypersensitive. Although the oral motor patterns of the two types of children are often similar, individual differences in oral sensory function should guide the selection of appropriate intervention methods.

Children with Hyposensitivity
and Hypotonicity

Children who are hyposensitive, and often hypotonic, receive reduced sensory feedback from the oral area and are less responsive in general to touch in and around the mouth. In infancy, such a child may be unsuccessful at breast feeding and may lack an adequate rooting and sucking reflex. With hypotonia, the proprioceptive mechanism is diminished and automatic oral responses are more difficult to elicit. Such a child is at risk nutritionally, as feeding may take longer and may proceed inefficiently. The child may have a lower arousal in general and may have poor endurance in nutritional sucking. The child may also have reductions in acuity of taste, smell, and touch pressure. These may contribute to indifference toward feeding (Morris & Klein, 1987).

Often children with low muscle tone, muscle weakness, diminished sensitivity, and poor endurance have specific oral motor problems. Mouth closure and lip seal are difficult to achieve. A stimulus on the tongue does not seem adequate to elicit mouth closure. Generally, controlled tongue motility is decreased resulting in a passive tongue; however, the tongue may exhibit wide excursions of poorly controlled movement. Typically the tongue falls back in the mouth into passive retraction.

As the infant matures and is given pureed food, more precise tongue movements are needed. The child with low tone, and hyposensitivity does not develop precise oral movement. With decreased tactile discrimination the lips and tongue are not stimulated to become active. Lateralization of the tongue is delayed, and subsequently the transfer of food from side to side of the mouth is inefficient, if not impossible. Often the jaw is unstable, and the child is unable to grade jaw movement. The child uses a primitive munching pattern that is inefficient for masticating hard, chewy foods.

Mature chewing involves midrange, rotary jaw movement and does not develop when the jaw is unstable. Cup drinking is another skill that requires jaw stability. The hypotonic and hyposensitive child tends to bite on the cup for stability and may lose liquid during the drinking process due to poor lip seal and poor mouth closure.

As the child is introduced to more textured food that is harder to chew, skills do not progress to adequately manage the food in the mouth. In children who are delayed in developing chewing, solid foods may be quite dangerous, as choking can occur. Thus, solid foods that do not dissolve, such as peanuts, raw carrots, or celery should not be offered (Morris, 1982). Hyposensitivity results in a child with primitive oral motor skill, who may demonstrate primitive but adequate patterns, which tend to limit the types rather than the amounts of foods consumed. Therapy and skill building tends to follow the normal developmental sequence.

Children with Hypersensitivity
and Hypertonicity

In hypersensitive children, oral problems may be more severe. These children may develop hypertonicity causing abnormal oral motor responses. Food intake is more difficult to manage and the child may be nutritionally at risk. This infant is often tactilely defensive and disorganized in feeding. A simple tactile input may cause a bite reflex or a tonic bite. Tongue thrust may be present as an exaggerated response to tactile or proprioceptive input. Abnormal reflexes may predominate when the child is inappropriately positioned (e.g., in extension) or when postural alignment is poor.

In a position of extension, the hypersensitive child usually demonstrates a suckle, characterized by extension-retraction of the tongue, rather than a suck, which includes an up and down tongue movement. The lip seal is incomplete on the nipple or the cup, and the lips may actually retract from the nipple. When abnormal reflexes and hypersensitivity interfere with the sucking, the infant may become disorganized. Oral movements becomes arrhythmical and sucking and swallowing lack coordination. The feeding process becomes frustrating and difficult for the infant and caretaker (Morris & Klein, 1987).

After sucking becomes a functional skill for the hypersensitive child, the cup and pureed food may be attempted. The tonic bite or the phasic bite release observed in infancy may re-emerge. Successful cup drinking requires that the infant be positioned with head and trunk stabilized. The first oral motor pattern observed with the cup or the spoon is one of suckling. Usually the tongue has a bunched up appearance and does not cup when drawing liquid into the month.

A prevalent behavior in the hypertonic child is exaggerated tongue protrusion. The tongue thrust or tongue retraction often interferes with mouth closure and interrupts the suckling sequence. Active lip movement to draw the food into the mouth is poorly developed. The lips may retract or purse, although this type of increased muscle tone is observed most often in older or severely involved children. The jaw moves in a wide range or a minimal range (as if clenching). In addition, uncoordinated jaw and tongue movement which may interfere with swallowing, and aspiration is possible. These uncontrolled behaviors are less likely to occur if the oral area is desensitized prior to feeding attempts.

INTERVENTION WITH A
SENSORY INVOLVED CHILD

The occupational therapist should consider four areas of sensory stimulation in feeding intervention for children with sensory deficits. These are discussed in the following order: (1) the environment; (2) handling prior to feeding; (3) positioning and handling during feeding; and (4) the sensory qualities of the food. All of these aspects of feeding can facilitate or hamper the child's feeding ability and oral sensory motor function.

The Environment

The environment refers to the general noise level, activity level and visual field provided by the environment. Feeding requires great concentration in children with sensory processing delays or deficits. The oral motor skill required in feeding is complex and the child is frequently stressed, due to the difficulties and frustrations previously experienced in feeding. A busy and noisy environment tends to distract and excite the child at a time when he or she needs concentration and organization.

Feeding is a high stress activity for both the hyposensitive and the hypersensitive child. The hyposensitive infant may resist oral feeding because it requires work and provides minimal pleasurable feedback. The hypersensitive child, who may want to eat, cannot organize and control his movements enough to do so efficiently. Given the stress levels of these children, the environment should promote calming with low levels of stimulation.

Children with disorganized or impaired feeding skills are entitled to a corner of the room or a quiet area. Noises and general activity should be kept to a minimum. Mealtime in classrooms may be facilitated with music. The best mealtime music is calm and relaxing, with one beat per second. The beat of the music simulates the rhythm of sucking in a normal infant (Morris & Klein, 1987). Good suggestions for the mother are to feed in a low light, quiet room using the child's favorite music box or her voice in a soothing manner.

Handling Prior to Feeding

The hyposensitive and hypotonic child often needs to be aroused. Although most infants become more alert and aroused prior to feeding when hungry, this increase in activity and tone may not occur in the hyposensitive child. Specific stimuli are used to increase the muscle tone and arousal state of the infant. A combination of vestibular and tactile stimuli can be a very powerful and effective method of arousal (Farber, 1982). However, alerting through rapid bouncing, rolling, and rubbing a child to facilitate an alert and aroused state prior to feeding may instead create stress and disorganization.

Handling should begin with simple and nonintrusive sensory stimuli which is increased gradually according to perceived readiness in the child. Simply moving an infant with hyposensitivity from a supine position into an upright position may achieve a bright, wide awake state. While upright, movement through space in the vertical plane may stimulate muscle tone. Alerting and increased muscle tone may be achieved in the child with hypotonicity by gently bouncing with adequate support to ensure that the child maintains neutral spinal alignment. When a child is in poor alignment, vestibular input does not effectively improve muscle tone, and may be disorganizing and uncomfortable for the child. Arrhythmical vestibular stimuli can be very arousing but can also be disorganizing.

Tactile stimulation is appropriate for both types of children and can be a preparatory activity that is arousing and organizing. Touch may be used to activate specific oral muscles in children with hypotonia and may decrease muscle tone in children with hypertonia. The therapeutic value of tactile stimulation is increased when the child participates in applying the stimulus. The goal is that he or she learn to apply the stimulus independently.

The oral area is approached systematically, first, by giving deep pressure to the chest to facilitate cervical flexion and assist the child in midline orientation. Next, symmetrical touch pressure may be provided to the face and mouth with the child's own hand assisting in stroking the cheeks and mandible. Light touch may be appropriate for children with hyposensitivity but should be avoided in children with hypersensitivity. Firm pressure is preferred, such that gum rubbing provides more proprioceptive than tactile input. Gum rubbing may be repeated on both sides, upper and lower gums, cautiously crossing the midline. The tongue, lips, and cheeks are usually very responsive to tactile input and an immediate motor response often results. Direct sensory motor interrelations tend to cause a rebound effect between sensory input and motor response.

Because the cranial nerves are intertwined in the brainstem and muscle spindles are prevalent (Kawamura & Morimotor, 1973) the effect of tactile and proprioceptive stimulation is likely to be immediate and in direct proportion to what is provided. The tactile input should be administered as a game and should include turn taking, frequent verbalization, and attention to the child's physical and verbal communication.

After rubbing the gums, rubbing the palate may be appropriate to desensitize or to enhance oral awareness. Sustained firm pressure to the midline of the palate may create an effect of general desensitization (Wilbarger, personal communication, 1987). Rubbing the finger wrapped in a towel across the tongue may improve tongue lateralization. Combining taste and touch often heightens sensory awareness, and the additional stimulus of taste with the pressure may have an alerting effect. The therapist's or caregiver's finger may be dipped in pureed food prior to applying deep pressure to gums. Use of a soft tooth brush on the gums may also activate oral structures. Rubber toys are often an acceptable stimulus for the child and can be guided with his or her participation onto sensitive areas of the mouth. During these sensory preparation activities careful attention and response to the child's cues are important.

Additional activities may be indicated in specific preparation of oral movement. Infants who persist in holding their neck in hyper-extension may need facilitation of neck elongation. Lengthening of neck extensors and activation of neck flexors are promoted through weight bearing and proprioceptive input with the child in a chin tucked position.

Handling During Feeding

The next consideration when working to improve feeding skills is positioning and handling during the actual intake of food. Correct posture and trunk alignment is essential for promoting the best oral motor skill in the child and for ensuring efficient suck and swallow so that food is not aspirated. In general an upright position is desired, although infants may be positioned in a semi-upright position. Eye contact is ideal, with the child able to view the therapist's or mother's face without chin jutting or neck hyper-extension.

The hypotonic child may collapse when brought into the completely upright position and this rounding of the trunk may compromise breathing. However, a reclined position facilitates extension which encourages tongue protrusion and mouth opening. A balance of flexion and extension is desired during feeding with emphasis on chin tuck, neck elongation, and trunk alignment. Neck elongation is facilitated by pressure upward and slightly forward behind the occipital lobe and the chin tuck is facilitated by input to the upper chest at the base of the neck and to the anterior chin. During feeding, the child should be completely supported so that trunk and head are stable and the child has optimal capability to control jaw, lips, and tongue. Oral movement takes great concentration and well established proximal stability. Midline, symmetrical positioning is also important to facilitate symmetrical oral movement.

To assist the child with hypotonia, jaw control may be used to promote stability. Jaw control is firm with consistent touch pressure under the base of the tongue, midway between the throat and the tip of the mandible. While in this position, the therapists hand responds to the child's movement, literally as an assist to jaw stability. The goal is to improve mouth closure and more isolated control of the tongue. In using jaw control, the therapist allows the child to guide her hand (Morris & Klein, 1987).

The hypersensitive infant is more likely to need swaddling or to need reinforcement of flexion and midline positions. Proximal stability should be provided, while allowing extremity movement (Harris, 1986). If the infant predominantly has uncontrolled, random movement, containment of extremities may assist the child in controlling oral movements. Jaw control can be beneficial for this child also, although the sensitive child may initially be uncomfortable with the tactile input, and the therapist must proceed slowly to improve the child's tolerance. With the hypersensitive child, the therapist must prioritize which forms of sensory input are most beneficial and which seem to cause more actual discomfort than assistance for the child.

Because children do not fall neatly into one category or another, no one or two positions and techniques work for each child. It is best to use a variety of positions that can be alternated given the fluctuating behavioral states and sensitivities of the infant.

Sensory Qualities of Food

The final form of intervention to be considered is the sensory quality of the child's food. The consistency and weight of the food determines the type of sensory input that it gives the child. Thin liquids are difficult to control and tend to trickle down both sides of the tongue. They are particularly difficult for the child with a bunched up or very flat tongue to control. Children with sensory processing deficits often have inefficient cheek and tongue action, and chewable foods that break apart into firm and diffuse pieces become lost and float into random directions rather than coming together to form a bolus. Once these foods are broken apart, it becomes impossible for the child to gather them together for chewing.

Softer foods or pureed foods easily form a bolus and can be more efficiently transported to the back of the mouth for swallowing. Pureed foods of smooth, thick consistency are definitely recommended for the child with a primitive suck-swallow pattern. However this sensory input is very limited and without progression to more textured, solid foods, chewing skills will not develop.

Solid foods provide more sensory input than pureed foods. The heavier, more cohesive bolus provides more tactile and proprioceptive sensation to the oral musculature. The heavier mass of solid food may facilitate a flattening and cupping of the tongue. Due to its physical properties, a bolus of solid food moves more slowly and the child has more time to control it. For the child with inadequate sensory processing, the additional proprioceptive input and the increased time to integrate that information may allow for more functional feeding. Examples of "heavier foods" are mashed potatoes or oatmeal.

The texture of the food effects the type of tongue, lip, and jaw movements observed. The hyposensitive child may exhibit more tongue and lip movement given a gritty, grainy, or lumpy food. Grapenuts or grits, for example, can be placed laterally to improve tongue lateralization. Crisp foods that dissolve, such as dried breakfast cereal, or gummy foods, such as chicken or bananas, are excellent for promoting chewing. Care must be taken in use of these types of food because the child may demonstrate a quick suck/swallow, without chewing, if the extra tactile input is too stressful for him. The hyposensitive child may not like crispy, grainy food and may require proceeding slowly from pureed to lumpier pureed to crispy, crunchy textures (Morris & Klein, 1987).

The hypersensitive child will also prefer smooth textured food of one consistency. Soft foods are important for this child and foods with lumps may not be tolerated. Perhaps the most difficult food type is that of a variety of consistencies such as vegetable soup or jello with fruit.

The texture and consistency of foods are selected according to the infant's developmental level and particular sensory motor problems. Chewy foods require more work. For example, using a piece of licorice may build muscle tone and help improve mouth closure when used prior to the meal. Highly textured, gritty foods may elicit more tongue movement and may help desensitize the mouth if they can be tolerated. Chewy and gummy foods hold together in a bolus for efficient swallow. Examples are chicken, dried fruit, and soft cheese.

Nutritional needs should never be compromised to build oral motor skills of the child. Consultation with a dietician or nutritionist is extremely beneficial when planning a diet or upgrading the kinds of foods that a child eats. A blender is helpful for providing a balanced diet of foods that are of appropriate consistency for the child. When liquids need to be thickened, wheat germ and jello should be considered, rather than baby cereal.

The nutritional value of the food and its texture and consistency should be carefully considered in planning a child's diet with his family. Often higher level oral motor skills may be elicited by varying the texture of the child's food. A variety of textures and tastes is always important to promote the child's tolerance of different foods and to ensure a balanced diet. The occupational therapist and parent should thoughtfully decide which foods are best for the infant, giving consideration to the nutritional needs of the infant, the food's consistency and texture, and the infant's and family's food preferences.

CONCLUSION

Infants with oral sensory deficits typically demonstrate primitive and deficient feeding skills and present a challenging problem to occupational therapists. Intervention should be carefully planned with the family, giving consideration to the environment during feeding and to the taste, texture, consistency, and nutritional value of the food offered. Strategies for improving oral motor skills include sensory stimulation to prepare the child for feeding and handling and positioning during feeding. Intervention that effectively enhances oral motor patterns and promotes positive and sensitive feeding interactions includes the parents' input and is guided by the infant's responses.

REFERENCES

Chusid, J. (1976). *Correlative neuroanatomy and functional neurology*. Los Altos, CA: LANGE Medical.

Farber, S. (1982). *Neurorehabilitation: A multisensory approach*. Philadelphia: Saunders Co.

Harris, M. (1986). Oral-motor management of the high-risk neonate. *Physical and Occupational Therapy in Pediatrics, 6*, (3/4), 231-254.

Kawamura, Y., & Morimoto, T. (1973). Neurophysiological mechanisms related to reflex control of tongue movement. In J. Bosma, (Ed.), *Oral sensation and perception: Development in the fetus and infant*. (pp. 206-217). Bethesda, MD: U.S. Dept. of Health, Education and Welfare, National Institutes of Health.

Morris, S. (1978). Selection of food and equipment for effective feeding therapy. In J. Wilson (Ed.), *Oral-motor function and dysfunction in children*. Chapel Hill, NC: Division of Physical Therapy, University of North Carolina, Chapel Hill.

Morris, S., & Klein, M. (1987). *Pre-feeding skills*. Tucson, AZ: Therapy Skill Builders.

Nowlis, G. (1973). Taste elicited tongue movements in human newborn infants: An approach to palatability. In J. Bosma, (Ed.), *Oral sensation and perception: Development in the fetus and infant*. (pp. 292-302). Bethesda, MD: U.S. Dept. of Health, Education, and Welfare, National Institutes of Health.

Rood, M. (1962). The use of sensory receptors to activate, facilitate and inhibit motor response, automatic and somatic in developmental sequence. In C. Sattely (Ed.) *Approaches to the treatment of patients with neuromuscular dysfunction*. Dubuque: W.C. Brown.

Rose, S. (1973). *The conscious brain*. New York: A.A. Knopf Co.

Tach, B. (1973). Morphologic zones of the human fetal lip. In J. Bosma, (Ed.), *Oral sensation and perception: Development in the fetus and infant*. (pp. 96-117). Bethesda, MD: U.S. Dept. of Health, Education, and Welfare, National Institutes of Health.

Clinical Management of Dysphagia in the Developmentally Disabled Adult

Margaret Stratton, MS, OTR/L

SUMMARY. As a member of a dysphagia team, the occupational therapist contributes a major part in both the assessment and treatment of swallowing disorders. Dysphagia referrals for developmentally disabled adults may range from aspiration and choking to rumination and refusal to eat. Using observations during mealtime, the therapist establishes a baseline for treatment planning. Related variables provide the focus and parameters of treatment. Although medical evaluations such as videoflouroscopy may provide expanded information, they are generally not critical in implementing an effective program.

The primary treatment objective, in most cases, is to develop active participation of the individual in the eating process. Most of these adults have never experienced "normal" mature eating patterns and may never achieve this level through treatment. The achievement of a functional level of eating will not only assist in maintaining the person's medical and nutritional status, but will facilitate a more positive mealtime experience.

The occupational therapist working in adult developmental disabilities is frequently challenged by referrals for the management of dysphagia (eating/swallowing dysfunction). Through direct clinical evaluation, the identification of specific oral-motor skills, related structural limitations, and environmental variables will assist in more accurately defining the problems. Based on the assessment

---

Margaret Stratton is the chief occupational therapist at J. N. Adam Developmental Disabilities Services Office in Perrysburg, NY.

The author wishes to acknowledge the administration, occupational therapy staff, speech pathology coordinator, and others at J. N. Adam for their roles in the development and growth of the dysphagia program.

143

information, treatment strategies are planned to develop active participation of the client in mealtime. Since eating is a dynamic process affected by many variables, communication with other team members and continued observation of and response to changes are essential.

ASSESSMENT

A comprehensive clinical assessment provides the direction for the design and implementation of an individualized dysphagia management program. Baseline information on eating skills and behavior helps to establish treatment objectives and criteria upon which progress can be measured. Environmental variables at mealtime, as well as non-mealtime information, assist the therapist in ensuring that the goals are realistic and obtainable.

Mealtime Assessment

The most significant aspect of the clinical dysphagia assessment is mealtime observation. If there are differences in mealtime settings (i.e., residential versus program), both sites should be included. The therapist's presence is often distracting and should be planned to cause the lest amount of disruption. By involving staff or family members in the evaluation, valuable information that is not apparent in the observation can be obtained (i.e., consistency of observed patterns and variables such as food preferences.) The basic components of a mealtime assessment include oral-motor function, position, muscle tone, primitive reflexes, type and presentation of food, utensils, and environment.

- *Oral-Motor Function*: Oral-motor function represents the oral or preparatory stage of swallowing. Since it is the only stage which is voluntary and directly observable and as it can influence subsequent stages, it is the primary focus in clinical management. The documentation of specific oral-motor patterns is completed using the Evaluation of Oral Function in Feeding (Stratton, 1981). Based on the scale of 0 "passive" to 5 "normal," each component of eating behavior is defined establishing a profile of strengths and needs. The individual's response is assessed differentiating spoon foods, liquids, and finger foods as appropriate to his existing diet. Function observed towards the midpoint of the meal is often most representative as a baseline since many individuals have difficulty in the initiation of oral-motor function and may also demonstrate fatigue towards the end of the meal. Any variations in patterns should be noted.

• *Position*: The individual's mealtime position is documented in relation to the "normal" model since subtle position changes often significantly affect treatment. Head and neck alignment, angle of head and trunk recline, and support for the upper and lower extremities are most essential.

• *Muscle Tone*: Any atypical muscle tone or fluctuation in tone is noted in relations to the observed eating patterns. It is important to differentiate tone and its effects from habitual patterns such as gravity-dependent "bird feeding." For example, head extension caused by extensor hypertonicity is often associated with jaw thrust or tongue thrust. Reduction in the tone will often reduce the related oral motor pattern. A habitual head extension pattern is not minimized through position changes and may have limited effect on eating.

• *Primitive Reflex Patterns*: Reflexes including the asymmetric and symmetric tonic neck, tonic labyrinthine, and associated reactions affect the individual's muscle tone and position. As with tone, these patterns must be identified to enable the therapist to relate them to eating patterns and modify them through position changes.

• *Presentation of Food/Liquid*: Whether the person feeds himself or is dependent on others, factors such as placement of food in the oral cavity, rate of eating, and time required to finish a meal should be documented.

• *Utensils*: The size of the utensil often affects food loss based on the amount of food which is most successfully manipulated in the oral cavity. The type of utensil (i.e., regular glass versus spouted cup) frequently changes the oral-motor response. These variables are noted in both initial and subsequent assessments to monitor their effect on eating.

• *Food*: Varied textures and consistencies of food often contrib-

ute to differences in oral-motor function. Individual food preferences of taste, texture, and temperature should be noted as
they are indicated through coughing, gagging, control of the
bolus, and refusal to eat/drink.

• *Environment*: Auditory and visual stimuli within the dining
room are reinforcing to some individuals while distracting to
others. The person's location in the room, response to surroundings, and level of interaction are noted in relation to success at mealtime.

Non-Mealtime Assessment

In addition to the completion of the mealtime assessment, occupational therapists also consider other factors such as oral structures, medical information, and a clinical history. They provide information on the limitations or rationale of a treatment plan which
may not be apparent in the direct assessment of eating skills.

• *Oral Structures*: In conjunction with a speech pathologist,
when available, an assessment of oral structures may assist in
defining a cause of eating difficulties. It also enables the therapist to recognize structural limitations in setting goals (i.e., lip
closure limited by the structure/alignment of mandible, max-
illa, and teeth).
  Included in a clinical evaluation of oral structures are: facial
tone; symmetry of head, neck, and face; presence and alignment of teeth; the status of the hard and soft palate; the size
and mobility of the tongue; nose versus mouth breathing; and
general level of oral sensitivity.

• *Medical Information*: From the client's record, information on
allergies, oral-facial surgery and scarring, gastro-intestinal
disorders, and respiratory complications is obtained. Medications may also relate to an eating difficulty including side effects of increased or decreased saliva, level of gag reflex, and
tardive dyskinesia.

• *Clinical History*: When available, early history of the client's
development and institutionalization may provide insights into
habitual patterns.

The combination of mealtime and non-mealtime information provides the occupational therapist with sufficient clinical data to develop a baseline of skills. It is also adequate, in most cases, to enable the therapist, in conjunction with other team members, to initiate an effective plan of treatment.

TREATMENT

Using assessment information, a profile of oral-motor function is developed as a baseline upon which changes can be monitored. Specific deficits are prioritized and addressed based on normal developmental sequences. Since many developmentally disabled adults are unable to generalize learned skills into new situations, an emphasis on direct mealtime interventions has been found to be most effective.

Mealtime treatment approaches include positioning, presentation of the food, utensils, and changes in diet. The primary objective is to develop an active participation in eating, or an increase in functional jaw, lip, and tongue movement.

- *Positioning*: The basis for any eating/swallowing program is a seating system which provides stability and alignment and is based on a "normal" model (Figure 1). Using assessment information of tone, reflexes, and current position, the therapist must bring the client in this position while minimizing the influence of abnormal muscle tone and primitive reflexes. Fixed orthopedic deformities may also prevent the client from achieving the optimal mealtime position. As the therapist works with other team members to reposition a client, other variables such as comfort and respiratory rate must be monitored. The final position must be effective not only for eating but for other aspects of the client's life as well.

  The closer the client's position is to this upright, slightly flexed posture of the head, neck, and trunk, the more potential there is to develop active oral-motor function. This forward head and neck position relates to the control of the bolus in the oral cavity during the initial stage of swallowing. As the client is reclined, the act of swallowing becomes increasingly gravity-dependent. The bolus, particularly thin foods or liquids, moves rapidly towards the pharynx without any time for oral sensation or manipulation. Individuals who have relied on this system over time not only increase the risk of aspiration, but also frequently develop passive jaw, lip, and tongue function.

The position of the head and neck most directly relates to a safe, effective swallow. By maintaining the head in an upright, slightly flexed posture, the client not only has optimal control of the bolus during the oral preparatory phase, but has protection of the airway as well. Although extension of the head and neck may be used by acute care patients as a com-

FIGURE 1. A "Normal" Model of Positioning

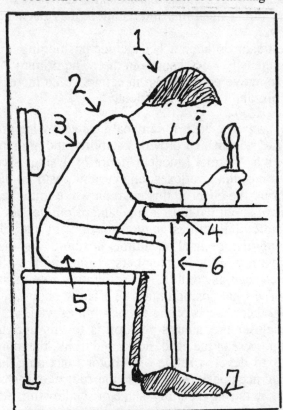

Description of Position	Function
1) <u>Head</u>--slightly flexed with chin in "tucked" position.	To provide optimal protection of the airway when swallowing.
2) <u>Shoulders</u>--slightly forward.	To provide relaxed neck/chest muscles related to breathing and swallowing.
3) <u>Trunk</u>--leaning slightly forward.	To provide optimal body alignment for digestion and respiration.
4) <u>Upper Extremities</u>-- weight bearing on elbows.	To provide stability of trunk and shoulders in maintaining an upright sitting posture.
5) <u>Hips</u>--flexed more than 90° and positioned at the back of the chair.	To provide the proper degree of pelvic tilt upon which to base a seated position.
6) <u>Knees</u>--flexed.	To properly position feet.
7) <u>Feet</u>--supported/ weight bearing.	To stabilize overall seated position.

pensatory technique to facilitate oral transit (Logemann, 1983), this may increase the risk of aspiration in a developmentally disabled individual. Persons who are unable to hold their breath should avoid this extended position due to the risk of unprotected airway during the swallow.

The same concept of head and neck position applies to individuals with a kyphosis. Bringing the head upright in relation to this should/trunk position also causes head/neck extension. For these individuals, the should position must be addressed initially in order to ensure proper alignment.

• *Presentation of Food*: Based on the information from the mealtime assessment, changes in the presentation of food may affect eating skills. Except for persons with a bite reflex, the utensil should contact the lips and remain in the oral cavity long enough to facilitate jaw and lip closure. Jaw control techniques (Mueller, 1972) may be used to physically assist this response. This technique should only provide guidance and not restrict the active jaw and tongue movement necessary for swallowing.

Firm, downward pressure one-third of the way back on the tongue inhibits increased tone and facilitates mobility. The pressure also provides additional sensory input to those who have been evaluated as having reduced oral sensitivity.

The rate of eating is crucial in the safe presentation of foods and liquids. Adequate time is needed following each reflexive swallow to allow all structures to return to their rest position before the next mouthful is introduced. When food occurs simultaneously in the oral and pharyngeal stages it significantly increases the risk of choking/aspiration and reduces the potential for active control. Individuals assessed as having poor oral sensitivity, delayed swallow, and reduced pharyngeal peristalsis are most vulnerable in this area.

• *Utensils*: Nosey cut-out glasses are used to ensure maintenance of a flexed head position while drinking. For individuals with delayed tongue response, teflon-coated or nylon spoons aid in providing downward pressure on the surface of the tongue without risk of injury to the tongue tissue. A tongue blade may assist for those persons with a sever bite reflex since it can be withdrawn from between the teeth without resistance.

Use of syringes and spouted cups should be avoided in the developmentally disabled since it bypasses the oral preparatory stage of swallow. In addition, prolonged use of these utensils often promotes a passive oral-motor response to eating.

• *Diet*: Based on the mealtime observations of the reaction to the taste, temperature, texture, and consistency of foods, the therapist must work in conjunction with the dietitian to make necessary changes. Subtle differences in the food directly influence the ability to sense, manipulate, and control the bolus. Some texture is necessary to facilitate lateral tongue movement and chewing. For those individuals with reduced oral sensitivity and limited tongue mobility, scattering textures (i.e., rice) may be difficult to manage. Increased thickness of foods may provide added sensation and control to those with a delayed swallow. The same consistency may increase fatigue in a person who exhibits excessive tongue movement when swallowing. Variables in taste may change eating patterns based on individual preferences. Cold foods may initially increase/facilitate an oral-motor response but may cause an inhibition of muscle activity over a prolonged period of time.

CONCLUSION

In dysphagia programs for the developmentally disabled adult, the occupational therapist plans an initial treatment approach based on an assessment of oral-motor function as it is influenced by other mealtime factors. Consideration must be given to areas such as deviations in oral structure, clinical history, and medical factors which may limit the potential to obtain specific objectives.

The treatment approach must continue as a dynamic process with ongoing observation/mealtime assessment of the person's response to position, diet, direct intervention, and environmental variables. The occupational therapist maintains communication with other team members to ensure an individualized, functional, and active approach to dysphagia management.

REFERENCES

American Occupational Therapy Association (1987). *Problems with Eating: Interventions for Children and Adults with Developmental Disabilities*. Maryland: AOTA.

Churney, L., Cantieri, C., and Pannell, J. (1986). *Clinical Evaluation of Dysphagia*. Rockville: Aspen Systems Corp.

Cromwell, F. (Ed.). Occupational Therapy for People with Eating Dysfunctions. *Occupational Therapy in Health Care*, *3*(2).

Farber, S. and Huss, J. (1974). *Sensorimotor Evaluation and Treatment Procedures for Allied Health Personnel*. Indiana: Indiana University Foundation.

Groher, M.E., (Ed.) (1984). *Dysphagia: Diagnosis and Management*. Massachusetts: Butterworth.

Logemann, J. (1983). *Evaluation and Treatment of Swallowing Disorders*. California: College Hill Press.

Perske, R., Clifton, A., McLean, B., and Stein, J. (1986). *Mealtimes for Persons with Severe Handicaps*. Baltimore: Paul H. Brooks.

Mueller, H.A. (1972). Facilitating Feeding and Pre-Speech. In Pearson, P.H., and Williams, C.E. (Eds.), *Physical Therapy Services in Developmental Disabilities*. Springfield: Charles C. Thomas.

Roueche, J.R. (1980). *Dysphagia: An Assessment and Management Program for the Adult*. Minneapolis: Sister Kenny Institute.

Stratton, M. (1981). Behavioral Assessment Scale of Oral Function in Feeding. *American Journal of Occupational Therapy*, *35*, 719-722.

Development and Implementation of a Dysphagia Program in a Mental Retardation Residential Facility

Carol A. Lust, MEd, OTR/L
Diane E. Fleetwood, BS, OTR/L
Elizabeth L. Motteler, MEd, CCC-SLP

SUMMARY. This paper describes the implementation of a dysphagia program in a residential mental retardation (MR) setting. Five program phases are presented describing the staff requirements, inservice and other procedures necessary to establish the program, the evaluation procedures, treatment approaches, and documentation

---

Carol A. Lust is Assistant Professor, Department of Occupational Therapy, School of Allied Health Sciences, East Carolina University, Greenville, NC 27858-4353. Carol received a master's degree in Special Education, specializing in the severely/profoundly handicapped, in 1986, and is presently responsible for the pediatric section of the Occupational Therapy curriculum at ECU. Diane E. Fleetwood is Staff Occupational Therapist, Caswell Center, North Carolina Division of Mental Health and Mental Retardation Services, Kinston, NC 28501. Diane has been involved in the clinical evaluation and treatment of swallowing disorders in a developmental disabilities setting since 1985. Elizabeth L. Motteler, Chief Speech Pathologist, The Pinnacle Care Rehabilitation Center, Wilmington, NC 28401, and Consulting Speech Pathologist Caswell Center, North Carolina Division of Mental Health and Mental Retardation Services, Kinston, NC 28501. Elizabeth has been involved in the clinical evaluation and treatment of swallowing disorders in an acute care/rehabilitation setting since 1985.

The authors wish to express their thanks to the staff administration and residents of the Caswell Center for their support and assistance in developing and implementing this program; to the Department of Speech-Language Pathology and Audiology, and the Department of Radiology of Pitt County Memorial Hospital; to June Urback for her help in preparing the manuscript; and to Dr. Robert Lust for editorial assistance in reviewing the manuscript.

patterns. Specific recommendations developed at Caswell to improve implementation of such a program with a residential, multi-handicapped population are discussed, and our initial results with evaluation procedures and therapeutic interventions in 56 residents are presented. In particular, a detailed analysis of 24 clients whose intervention was based on videofluoroscopic examination are also presented.

INTRODUCTION

Dysphagia, or difficulty with swallowing, is currently gaining interest due to its increasingly identified relationship to medical problems frequently encountered in the multihandicapped, mentally retarded (MR) resident population. It has been reported that the leading cause of death in the institutionalized, severely retarded population is asphyxia (Carter & Jancear, 1984) and upper respiratory infection, presumably due to aspiration of food (Carter & Jancear, 1983; McCurley, Mackay, & Scally, 1972). In fact, at Caswell (total resident population 900), 28 of 254 multihandicapped residents (approximately 1 of every 10) have been hospitalized with admitting diagnoses directly related to feeding deficits (Table 1). Consistent with the previous report, seventy-five percent of these admitting diagnoses include aspiration pneumonia.

Swallowing impairments may be present secondary to anatomical

Table I.

Admitting Diagnoses in 28 Residents Hospitalized in 1985 with Problems Related to Feeding Deficits.

Aspiration pneumonia	21
Dehydration	2
Weight Loss	1
Chronic upper respiratory infection	6
Other	3

Note: Several of the 28 residents were admitted with multiple diagnoses.

damage in the oral, pharyngeal or esophageal areas. Also, the normal physiology of the oral-pharyngeal swallowing process may be disrupted (Logemann, 1987). Neurological and neuromuscular diseases, head and neck injuries, local structural lesions, cancer, gastrointestinal disorders, and birth defects may produce dysphagic symptoms. Therapeutic approaches for relief of these symptoms have been largely directed towards rehabilitating patients with acquired dysphagia secondary to acute disease processes (Logeman, 1983). However, in the multihandicapped MR resident, dysphagic symptoms are more often related to inherited rather than acquired abnormalities, and little information is available about the diagnostic or therapeutic approach to dysphagia in this population. Therefore, this article was written to report our experience in developing and implementing a dysphagia program with the multihandicapped population of a residential MR facility. Five program phases are presented; Phase I: identify and train the swallowing team; Phase II: form development and staff in-service training; Phase III: bedside evaluation and observation; Phase IV: videofluoroscopic examination (VFSE); and Phase V: therapeutic implementation. Modifications to evaluation, therapy, and assessment procedures necessitated by the special characteristics of this population are described, as are our initial results with 56 residents in the Caswell swallowing program.

PHASE I:
IDENTIFY AND TRAIN THE SWALLOWING TEAM

Implementation of a dysphagia program initially requires additional professional staff training to develop the necessary levels of advanced expertise. At Caswell Center, the following professionals formed the swallowing team: an occupational therapist, a speech-language pathologist, a dietitian, a physician, and a nurse. Team members should be able to provide vital information in the management of a resident with a swallowing disorder and have an interest in this aspect of therapy. In addition, these team members should have at least one year of experience with the multihandicapped, mentally retarded population.

Possible roles for each swallowing team member are described as follows. The Occupational Therapist evaluates each resident and recommends or provides any adaptive dining equipment, positioning devices, or oral-motor facilitation treatment programs that may be indicated. The Speech Pathologist evaluates a resident's present level of communicative functioning and is directly involved in the re-education of the muscle groups of the oral cavity and larynx. The dietician evaluates each resident's nutritional status and fluid intake, assists in development and carrying out special diet recommendations. The attending physician is responsible for the primary medical care of the resident and coordinates total medical and surgical management. The team nurses, through physician orders, have direct responsibility for monitoring the resident's medical and nutritional status, and are directly involved in both oral and non-oral intake (Groher, 1984).

One member of the swallowing team, regardless of professional background should be identified as the swallowing therapist. The swallowing therapist should obtain advanced training in the evaluation and treatment of swallowing disorders. Training should include anatomy and physiology of normal and abnormal swallowing patterns, observation of videofluoroscopic evaluations and swallowing intervention planning. The above information could be acquired by attending a three day course, although attending such a workshop would depend upon the support and financial resources of your facility. However, lack of access to such a concentrated course could significantly delay the training process and, therefore, initiation of the swallowing program would be hindered. At Caswell Center several Occupational Therapists and Speech Pathologists have attended Logemann workshops. Caswell Center presently has four swallowing teams.

Once educated, the swallowing therapist(s) should visit other established programs to obtain experience, share knowledge, exchange ideas, and develop support systems within the surrounding geographical area. If multiple swallowing teams are planned, one swallowing therapist should be designated to assume a leadership role in coordinating the development of the swallowing program and the teams involved. The swallowing coordinator serves as a resource to each team and swallowing therapist for the entire program. This individual should be present in each evaluation. The coordinator keeps each team updated on current dysphagia developments and has a working knowledge of swallowing disorders throughout the facility. By reviewing all of the dysphagia studies, the swallowing coordinator develops expertise in diagnostics evaluation.

Upon completion of these steps, the team should draft formal recommendations and procedures for implementing the swallowing program. It is important that this occur as the final step so that the swallowing coordinator will have the necessary base of knowledge to support, discuss and implement the program. The program proposal should outline steps to (1) identify residents who may be appropriate for evaluation, (2) refer residents for evaluation, (3) evaluate each resident's dysfunction by the swallowing team, and (4) implement the recommended treatment procedures. Within each of these areas, step by step instructions should be provided, and should define the responsibilities of each swallowing team member in every phase of the evaluation. The procedural proposal should then be presented for formal institutional, administrative board and medical service review for final approval. At Caswell Center the initial phase, from team identification, through training and final approval, took approximately 11 to 12 months to complete.

PHASE II:
FORM DEVELOPMENT
AND STAFF IN-SERVICE TRAINING

To insure efficient staff communication, two forms were developed: a referral form and a swallowing/dining protocol form (see appendix A & B). Both forms were developed by Caswell's swallowing therapists based upon examples provided by other established swallowing programs within the state. Both forms require administrative approval prior to utilization. Obtaining administrative approval greatly improved staff acceptance and use of these forms when the swallowing program began. In addition, the swallowing/dining protocol form required additional approval by the institutional forms committee for inclusion in the resident's chart. Detailed aspects of this form are discussed further in PHASE 5 (below).

The referral form contains the resident's identifying information, current medical diagnoses, and a description of the swallowing problem(s), a checklist of mealtime behavioral observations, the current diet, and adaptive dining equipment. This provides vital information to the swallowing therapist prior to evaluation of the resident by the swallowing team. As the next step, the swallowing team should provide in-service training for all staff members. General information about the new dysphagia program, and specific details regarding procedural aspects of the program should be discussed. This includes correct use of the newly developed referral form.

For maximum effect, separate in-services were specifically geared to each level of staff that were or are to be involved. These levels were loosely defined as administrative, department head, professional and support staff. To facilitate exposure, in-service programs were often scheduled during monthly administrative/departmental meetings. At each in-service, a swallowing therapist was present, along with a second member of the swallowing team. Each in-service participant was given a copy of the administratively approved protocol on the swallowing program and a copy of the referral form. It was explained that the referral could be initiated by the physician or the resident's habilitation team, either at the yearly team meeting or during an interim meeting. This completed referral form should then be forwarded to the swallowing team. A videotape highlighting both normal and abnormal videofluoroscopic studies is a highly recommended component of the in-service program. Each in-service meeting usually lasted approximately 30 to 45 minutes, depending on the level of discussion encountered.

The swallowing team(s) should allocate approximately two to three months to develop the necessary forms, provide in-service programs for the entire staff, and complete phase II. This time frame obviously will vary according to the size of the facility.

PHASE III:
BEDSIDE EVALUATION AND OBSERVATION

Ideally, each swallowing disorder referral should be evaluated using the bedside evaluation in conjunction with a videofluoroscopic examination (VFSE). The specific basis for referral to the dysphagia program is provided in Table 2. We recognize that the swallowing therapist is not able to assess the pharyngeal stage of swallowing in a bedside evaluation. Coughing is not a reliable indicator of aspiration tendencies, and Logemann reports as many as 40% of the swallowing disorders involving an aspiration component may not be detected without VFSE. However, there are practical limitations. Due to the technical, fiscal, and professional constraints inherent to many residential MR facilities, VFSE of each swallowing disorder referral is usually not possible. Therefore, we tend to use the bedside evaluation to investigate possible alternative approaches and as a means to screen referrals for further assessment using VFSE as well.

The bedside evaluation contains the resident's medical diagnosis, method of food intake, drug history, respiratory status, level of alertness, ability to follow directions, hydration and nutritional status, any dietary restrictions, and an assessment of anatomical defects. Sensory testing of the lips, tongue, palate, pharynx, and larynx as they pertain to speech, mastication, salivation and/or

Table 2.

Reason for Referral of 50 Residents to the Dysphagia Program, from Janaury 1986 to May 1988.

Choking	25
Vomiting	5
Weight Loss	4
Coughing	16
Aspirtion pneumonia	6
Delay or absent swallow	8
Recurrent upper respiratory infection	1
Other	7

Note: Several of the 50 residents were referred with multiple problems.

swallowing should be performed. Motor testing of speech and swallowing function should also be included.

In addition, the multihandicapped nature of the resident requires several alterations to the "standard" bedside evaluation. Specifically, the past and present oral facilitation therapy programs, the adaptive dining equipment, and any diet texture changes that have been attempted must be considered. Also, the resident's fatigue level and any position options that may have been tried must be taken into account. Finally, due to the resident's mental and cognitive level, several aspects of the "standard" bedside evaluation may not be possible. For example, volitional control is often absent, and this is a necessary component in the assessment of speech and swallowing function. In addition, voluntary initiation of tongue movements is often not possible, and the swallowing therapist must rely heavily on direct observations during an actual meal.

In assessing methods of food intake, it is extremely beneficial to request that the resident's primary caregiver assist in feeding or independently feed the resident. This allows the swallowing therapist to observe firsthand the resident's optimum functioning level and to establish a baseline of current skills. After the baseline has been established, the swallowing therapist should attempt to feed every resident and use therapeutic approaches to improve quality of feeding. Several approaches, such as a change in the resident's head position, food presentation patterns, or perhaps changes in diet textures could be attempted. These trial techniques are very helpful in determining the appropriate recommendations.

It is our policy to complete the bedside evaluation within ten working days of referral. Once completed, the swallowing team recommends one of two approaches. These are (1) continued oral feeding in conjunction with a designated oral-motor program, and (2) further analysis using VFSE. At our institution, the rate of assignment to each of these approaches, including several of the variations in oral feeding approaches, is shown in Table 3.

Once the swallowing team has completed assessment and recommendations, the swallowing therapist writes a swallowing evaluation report. It is our policy that the written report should be submitted within 10 working days following completion of the evaluation. The report is then submitted to the resident's physician for ap-

Table 3.

Recommendations Made for 50 Residents Following Bedside Evaluation

Videoflouroscopy	24
Diet texture change	11
Oral motor exercises	11
Dining procedures	10
Supervision	11
Adaptive dining equipment	12
Alternative feeding	3
Data collection	3
Other	3
No recommendations made, follow-up in 6 months	2

Note: Several residents received multiple recommendations

proval/disapproval and distributed to the habilitation team. At Caswell Center, the process of referral, evaluation, and initial recommendation (Phase III) can require as much as one month to complete.

PHASE IV:
VIDEOFLUOROSCOPIC EXAMINATION

Our bedside evaluation procedures have been successful in directing 44% (Table 3), of the swallowing disorder referrals to treatment regimens without the use of additional VFSE. Therapeutic plans are specifically tailored to the individual resident, and a detailed discussion of these is beyond the scope of the present article. Instead, the present discussion will concentrate on the special requirements necessary to complete the recommended additional assessment successfully using VFSE (56%, Table 3).

162 Developmental Disabilities: A Handbook for Occupational Therapists

Once the VFSE recommendation is approved, the swallowing therapist schedules an appointment at the nearest regional rehabilitation center or acute care facility possessing a radiology unit, and forwards a copy of the swallowing evaluation. Lag times of one month may frequently be encountered in scheduling this exam. Additional constraints on the regional center are that hospital liability and restrictions on privileges usually require that the regional center also have a dysphagia program, with a swallowing therapist that can assist in the VFSE and its interpretation.

Staff necessary for the study include the radiologist, the regional rehabilitation center's swallowing therapist, and the residential MR facility's swallowing therapist. In addition, an occupational therapist and the resident's primary caregiver may also be needed. The occupational therapist may be needed to assist in proper positioning, and the caregiver may be quite helpful during the actual feeding portion of the study.

In general, VFSE refers to the radiographic study used to examine the oral preparatory, oral, pharyngeal, and upper esophageal stages of swallowing. More precisely, dysphagia referrals are commonly assessed using a modified barium swallow (MBS). This analysis utilizes a standard amount of liquid barium, barium paste, and a barium coated cookie to assess the speed of the swallow, and any motility problems in the oral cavity, larynx or pharynx. In addition, the etiology and timing of aspiration, if present, can also be identified (Logemann, 1983). However, it should also be noted that several modifications to the usual MBS may be required to successfully complete a VFSE with a multihandicapped individual. Alterations in positioning, feeding utensils, and manner of food presentation may all be necessary.

Physical deformities, fluctuating muscle tone, and abnormal primitive reflex patterns can create difficulties with the upright sitting position commonly employed in MBS procedures. We have found that using an infant seat is most helpful in normalizing postural tone and making the resident as comfortable as possible. To maintain the proper head position, velcro strapping and pillows may be necessary. That failing, the resident's head sometimes must be manually stabilized in the therapeutic feeding position.

Different types of adaptive feeding equipment may also be required to complete a MBS in a mutlihandicapped individual. A medicine dropper, a syringe, a medicine cup, a cut-out cup, and different sized nipples for infant bottles may be needed to present the liquid barium for ingestion. To successfully present the barium paste, the swallowing therapist should determine the correct sized spoon, and determine whether or not it should be rubber coated. Whenever possible, the resident's own adaptive dining equipment should be used during the study.

A MBS in an individual that is not multihandicapped involves the study of swallows using substances varying in size. However, the multihandicapped individual is never presented with food of varying size. Because the MR multihandicapped resident usually does not have adequate lip closure or cannot follow verbal directions, the food portion is always a 1/3 of a teaspoon (Logemann, 1987). Caswell's specific recommendations concerning food presentation to the multihandicapped undergoing MBS includes spoon presentation of the barium paste to the posterior section of the tongue. Also, mixing the paste with preferred food items like chocolate pudding or applesauce may improve success with these procedures. In addition, the resident's oral motor control may be so poor that the final substance (the barium cookie) portion of the test may have to be omitted. Finally, the resident's comprehension limitations and short attention span may restrict the effort to determine the resident's optimal swallowing ability. The resident may not comprehend instructions that are needed for safe oral intake. If the primary caregiver is needed to assist with the feeding, care must be taken to insure that good radiation safety procedures are followed. The entire procedure (waiting, registration, positioning, etc.) may require as much as two hours to complete, although the actual radiographic time may be as little as 5-10 minutes.

Immediately following the MBS, the radiologist and the evaluating swallowing therapist review the videotape. The level of involvement (Cherney, Cantieri & Pannell, 1986) and areas of dysfunction are identified and appropriate treatment recommendations are made (Figure 1). These findings are summarized in a preliminary report and given to the MR residential facility's swallowing therapist the same day. The formal report is completed and mailed to the residential facility within two weeks. To complete this phase,

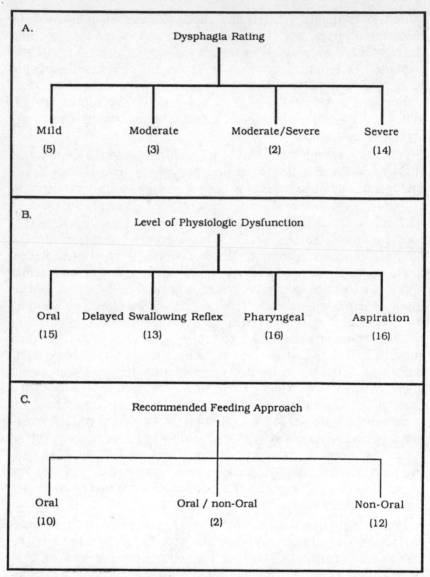

FIGURE 1. Summary of findings from 24 videofluoroscopic procedures referred from the Caswell Center, including the severity of involvement (Panel A), the physiologic nature of the underlying dysfunction (Panel B), and the recommended therapeutic feedings approach (Panel C). Note that evaluations commonly cited several physiologic disorders.

from initial VFSE referral, through scheduling and completing the MBS and formulating the therapeutic recommendation, may take two weeks to four weeks.

PHASE V:
THERAPEUTIC IMPLEMENTATION

After appropriate approval of the recommendations (oral versus non-oral intake, therapy techniques, or compensatory techniques), the swallowing therapist should proceed to implement the treatment recommendations. The first step in implementation at Caswell Center is to document the intended treatment plan on the swallowing/dining protocol form and place it in the resident's chart (sample provided in the appendix). The form contains a section for oral motor exercises, thermal stimulation procedures, and dining procedures including current diet textures, adaptive dining equipment, and specific serving procedures. This form is completed by the swallowing therapist and information included is based upon recommendations developed by the swallowing team. We have found that in some cases all three sections are completed and in other cases only one section is completed. The form is updated as needed by the swallowing therapist, depending upon the resident's status.

At the present time, our swallowing therapists are unable to provide direct swallowing therapy due to other job duties and responsibilities. Thus, the second step in implementation is to train the staff from the resident's unit to properly implement the recommended treatment and therapy procedures. This is accomplished by scheduling intensive in-service training for the staff working with the resident. The staff are given a copy of the swallowing/dining protocol and the swallowing therapist verbally explains all of the information. This is followed by hands-on demonstration of the techniques using staff and/or the resident. The swallowing therapist ensures that each staff person has a clear understanding of the information, and can implement these procedures effectively. Training the staff at this level takes approximately one week.

Upon completion of the formal training, successful implementation of the swallowing program is insured by following a schedule of gradually decreasing involvement by members of the swallowing team. During the first two weeks of implementation, the swallowing therapist should feed the resident once daily. During the third week the professional assistant (such as a COTA or LPN) should serve the resident once daily, and by the fourth week, the primary caregiver should assume complete responsibility for implementing the resident's swallowing program. This schedule allows the swallowing therapist time to monitor program effectiveness and make any needed modifications in the swallowing/dining protocol. Currently, therapy procedures (oral motor exercise and thermal stimulation) are implemented seven days per week, three times daily, for approximately 10-15 minutes prior to mealtime. The staff members then proceed directly to mealtime dining procedures. This insures that the resident receives maximum benefit from the therapy and that oral-intake is as safe as possible.

Documentation of the swallowing/dining protocol procedures and progress should follow this schedule: the swallowing therapist should document observation of the primary caregiver and resident at a different meal each day for the first two weeks, progressing to once every two weeks for one month, and if all goes well, to monthly observations by the swallowing therapist. Formal quarterly reports on the swallowing program should be written for each resident. This report should contain general observations, consistency of program implementation, caregiver's input regarding the resident's performance, the resident's tolerance to the program, meal intake, weight gain (or loss), any change in the frequency of coughing/choking episodes, and the resident's tolerance to current diet texture.

Treatment strategies in a multihandicapped MR population often challenge the swallowing therapist. Common problems which hinder treatment approaches are the resident's low cognitive level, resistance to oral-facilitation techniques, and the persistence of abnormal oral-motor skills.

Only two of the therapy techniques usually recommended for swallowing disorders are appropriate for our population. The first are oral-motor exercises which serve to improve the speed, strength and range of lip and tongue movements, permitting better bolus control during the voluntary stage of the swallow. The second is thermal stimulation, which is beneficial in heightening the awareness of the swallow (Logemann, 1983).

Nonetheless, we have developed modifications to the conventional approach that produces successful treatment intervention for the MR resident. For oral-motor exercise programs we have used lollipops, frozen caramel candy on a stick, or popsicles to accomplish lip and tongue exercises. These techniques work extremely well with lower functioning residents who cannot imitate or perform volitional oral-motor exercises. The types of food used in these exercises are also excellent positive reinforcers to the resident. We have found that flexible fish tank tubing works just as well as licorice sticks for improving tongue control of the bolus, with the advantage of minimal cost and easy accessibility.

During thermal stimulation therapy, frozen lemon glycerin swabs, and frozen nonbreakable drink stirrers are used instead of laryngeal mirrors. The laryngeal mirrors are expensive for the institution and dangerous to the resident that exhibits pica behaviors (consuming inedible objects). Finally, we have eliminated possible judgment errors or new staff error by providing each resident with an infant size spoon to ensure that each bite of food is limited to 1/3 teaspoon. As more residents are evaluated for swallowing disorders, and therapy is recommended, swallowing therapists must continue to be creative and innovative in the application of "conventional" treatment modalities to the multihandicapped MR population.

CONCLUSION

We have described our experience with the logistics of developing and implementing a dysphagia program in a MR, multihandicapped resident population. Alternatives to including videofluoroscopic examination (VFSE) in the assessment of each patient were described. In those patients requiring videofluoroscopy, the modifications to standard techniques that were necessary to successfully complete this procedure were described. In our experience, fifty percent of the residents requiring VFSE to assess dysphagic symptoms were ultimately recommended to a non-oral feeding program. In oral feeding programs, oral-motor exercises and thermal stimulation (with several modifications) were the most commonly recommended therapies. At this stage our results are largely qualitative. However, preliminary analysis of the impact of the swallowing program in 24 residents initially evaluated using VFSE is as follows (Figure 2).

Six residents had to be excluded from analysis due to the complicated nature of their medical course and because the relation of the medical problem to a feeding deficit could not be clearly estab-

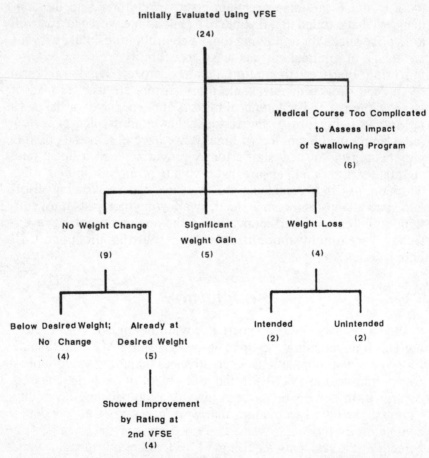

FIGURE 2. Preliminary analysis of the impact of the swallowing program in the 24 residents initially evaluated. Using VFSE.

lished. Of the remaining 18, 5 (28%) showed improvement as indicated by significant weight gain. Four residents exhibited a weight loss, but half of these were expected from medical orders to reduce intake. The unintended weight loss remains unexplained. Nine residents (50%) showed no weight change, but more than half (5) of these were already within the desired weight range. Of these 5 residents, 80% showed improvement as rated during a follow-up VFSE. Thus, between positive weight gain and improved VFSE rating, 50% (9/18) of the most severely involved residents demonstrated improvement after enrollment in the swallowing program.

We are encouraged to note that even in the most severely involved subset (those requiring VFSE to assess), preliminary review indicates that fully one-half have shown improvement following placement in the swallowing program. These results are preliminary, and are focused on the implementation of the program. The ultimate impact of such a program on issues such as the number of choking episodes, feeding time needed by the care giver, or cost effectiveness remains to be established in our institution.

On the basis of our demonstrated need, and early results following initiation of a swallowing program, we would recommend that similar swallowing programs be considered in other residential MR facilities. In implementing a swallowing program details for quantitative evaluation of program impact should be established from the beginning. Swallowing team members must be prepared to be innovative in adapting programs to the particular needs of their resident population.

REFERENCES

Carter, G., Jancar, J. (1983). Mortality in mentally handicapped: Fifty-year survey at stoke park group hospitals. *Journal of Mental Deficiency Research, 27,* 143-156.

Carter, G., Jancar, J. (1984). Sudden deaths in mentally handicapped. *Psychology Medicine, 14,* 691-695.

Cherney, L. R., Cantieri, C. A., Pannell, J. J. (1986). *Clinical evaluation of dysphagia.* Rockville: Aspen.

Donner, M. W. (1986). Editorial. *Dysphagia, 1,* 1-2.

Groher, M. E. (1984). *Dysphagia diagnosis and management.* MA: Butterworth.

Logemann, J. A. (1983). *Evaluation and treatment of swallowing disorders.* San Diego: College-Hill Press.

Logemann, J. A. (1987, October). *The role of the speech language pathologist in the management of dysphagia*. Paper presented at the Evaluation and Treatment of Dysphagia: A Workshop. Chicago, IL.

McCurley, R., Mackay, D. N., Scally, B. G. (1972). Life expectation of mentally subnormal under community and hospital care. *Journal of Mental Deficiency Research, 16*, 57-66.

Appendix A
CASWELL CENTER
REFERRAL FOR SWALLOWING EVALUATION

Date:_____

Referring Source:_____   Name:_____

Functioning Level:_____   Case No.:_____

Date of Onset of Problem:_____   DOB:_____DOA:_____

                                                                 Unit/Div.:_____

Medical Diagnoses:_____
_____

Brief description of problem:_____
_____
_____

Current Diet:_____

Adaptive Feeding Equipment:_____

Please answer:
  Can the resident follow simply gestural/verbal commands?_____
                              Verbal_____   Nonverbal_____
  Any coughing during dining?_____   Any choking during dining?_____
  Any recent unexplained weight loss?_____
  Is there a history of chronic respiratory problems?_____
  Is there a persistent mucus build-up or secretion?_____
  Are any specific foods or liquids more difficult for the resident? (Please
    list):_____
_____
  Does the resident self-feed?_____
  Is the resident ambulatory or non-ambulatory?_____
  Are there any behavior problems; (if so, please describe and note if a
    program exists)_____
_____
_____

Please enter name:

    Social Worker:_____
    Speech-Language Pathologist:_____
    Occupational Therapist:_____
    Dietitian:_____
    DT Advocate:_____
    Physician:_____
    RN:_____
    MRHC II:_____

Appendix B

Caswell Center

NORTH CAROLINA
DIVISION OF MENTAL HEALTH
AND MENTAL RETARDATION SERVICES

SWALLOWING/DINING PROTOCOL

EVALUATOR:_____

DATE:_____

I. ORAL-MOTOR EXERCISES:

II. THERMAL STIMULATION:

III. DINING PROCEDURES:
    A. DIET -

    B. ADAPTIVE DINING UTENSILS -

    C. PROCEDURES -

Form No. DMH MRP 4-10-78   TEAM PROGRAM GOALS & PLAN
07-145-1187

Pre-Vocational Programming
in a Pediatric Skilled Care Facility

Jeanne E. Lewin, MS, OTR/L

SUMMARY. This article describes a pre-vocational program that was developed in a private residential skilled care pediatric facility, under the guidance of an occupational therapy consultant. This "Special Training Program" was designed to meet the needs of the few higher functioning adolescents and young adults residing within the facility who did not participate in daily community school programs.

This paper presents the philosophical issues related to developing a pre-vocational program; the criteria for selecting program participants; the program structure (implementation details, work sample selection, production rate data records, program supervision, participant remuneration, physical set-up and start-up costs); and an evaluation of the benefits and disadvantages of the program following one year of the Special Training Program's initiation date.

INTRODUCTION

With an increasing number of occupational therapists being utilized as consultants to large residential facilities serving clients with developmental disabilities, the therapist must assist the facility staff in developing strategies to meet residents' needs. Periodically those strategies call for initiating a new program within the facility, which may require additional funds and a reorganization of full-time staff

Jeanne E. Lewin is currently Clinical Supervisor of Pediatrics, Occupational Therapy Department, Rehabilitation Institute of Chicago, Chicago. She also maintains a limited private practice.

Copies of the Resident Pre-Vocational Participant Selection Evaluation and other forms related to the training program can be obtained for $10.00 by writing Jeanne E. Lewin, 894 St. Andrews Way, Frankfort, IL 60423.

responsibilities and commitments. This article describes a pre-vocational program, "Special Training Program" (STP), that was developed in a pediatric skilled care residential facility by the author, referred to in this paper as "the consultant." Steps taken in the development of this program may be applied to a variety of day school or residential facilities. Specific details regarding the participant selection process, development and evaluation of the work sample and work-related behaviors are provided.

The first part of this paper will highlight the mechanics and the development of the STP. The second part will present a critique of the pre-vocational program following one year of operation in the pediatric skilled care facility.

SETTING AND POPULATION

This pre-vocational program was developed by an occupational therapy consultant in a privately funded, 128 bed, skilled care, pediatric residential facility for children from birth to 21 years of age. The Special Training Program was designed to meet the needs of the few higher functioning adolescent and young adult residents. These individuals did not participate in daily community school programs outside of the facility. The functional level of a majority of the residents is in the severe to profound range of cognitive and physical abilities. The full time therapy department at the facility consists of four certified occupational therapy assistants (COTA's), six Therapy Aides, and one Speech and Language Pathologist.

PROGRAM RATIONALE

Background

Adulthood is a time when one undertakes a life-task role with an increased emphasis on work responsibilities and related behaviors and basic finance and budgeting issues (Hopkins & Smith, 1983). Play becomes relaxation and recreation during the adult years and acts as a supportive component to the worker role (Kielhofner, Burke, & Igi, 1980).

For the majority of institutionalized mentally retarded individuals, the transition from adolescence to adulthood is generally not accompanied by an increase in personal responsibilities concomitant with one's chronological maturation. However, through special occupational guidance and programming by health care providers, this population may have the opportunity to be nurtured in developing appropriate work behaviors and physical and manual skills necessary for employment outside of the residential facility. The STP was designed to provide a milieu in which older adolescents and young adults in a residential facility could functionally develop such work related behaviors and skills.

Vocational education is a major segment of American education. Public Law 94-142, The Education for All Handicapped Children Act of 1975, and Public Law 94-482, the Vocational Education Amendment of 1976, explicitly recognize the special needs of handicapped individuals. Each law addresses a complimentary area of concern as well as providing funding support for facilities to provide service in these areas of need. Public Law 94-482 specifically references The Education for All Handicapped Children Act, requires conformity with it and states that federal grants be provided to states for support of vocational educational programs for individuals with special education needs (Weisgerber, Dahl, & Appleby, 1981).

Transitional programming by educators from the academic/ school environment to the work place are being emphasized for those students who are approaching secondary school graduation. In several states, some special educators serve as vocational adjustment coordinators and have duties similar to those of a vocational counselor (Brolin, 1976).

Based on the assumption that occupational therapy must be "occupation" (Kielhofner et al., 1980) and the assertion that occupational therapy is directed towards enabling humans to fulfil their need for occupation (Reilly, 1962), a therapeutic program must embody purposefulness, challenge, accomplishment and satisfaction. It is therefore natural that the occupational therapist who consults to a facility serving the mentally retarded/multiplehandicapped will focus the therapy services on pre-vocational assessment and programming. In the STP, the author acted as developer, facilitator and partial implementor for the program.

Purpose

The purpose of developing the STP was twofold. The first and foremost purpose was to expose the residents to and give them an opportunity to establish work-related behaviors. Work-related behaviors are defined here as those behaviors that are critical for success in a vocational setting. Attendance and punctuality, accuracy and speed of work, neatness, motivation, and reaction to constructive criticism are examples of work-related behaviors (Scott, Ebbert, & Price, 1986; Stephens, 1978; Wehman, Kregel, & Barcus, 1985).

The second purpose of the STP was to orient the participant to the world of work while addressing specific work deficiencies and maladaptive behaviors which deter the participant from obtaining work. "Work" is the primary treatment media in a work adjustment program. Don Brolin, in his book *Vocational Preparation of Retarded Citizens*, states that work adjustment skills must be developed in the mentally retarded individual before formal work evaluation efforts may be conducted (Brolin, 1976, 1982).

Upon reviewing the programs of these older residents who ranged in age from 15 to 21 years, the consultant learned that much of their occupational therapy programming fell into one of three categories: (1) Activities of Daily Living Skills, primarily dressing skills related to fastenings; (2) self-feeding skills; and (3) fine motor tasks which enhance their manipulative abilities. These programs were generally implemented on a one-to-one basis by the Certified Occupational Therapy Assistant (COTA) on a rather inconsistent schedule. There also appeared to be a limited opportunity outside of the therapy session of these residents to reinforce the skills practiced in therapy.

This led to consideration of a more functional as well as motivational program for residents to achieve the same goals and be provided on a consistent schedule; such a program could be designed to foster adaptive skills that would have a significant impact on the future of these older individuals outside of the facility. The guiding question for this program was whether these residents currently and probably destined to remain in the facility for life could be given preparation in skills which might lead to future placements for them.

Since this particular facility is a pediatric home, there was some urgency to develop a means by which these older residents might acquire skills that would foster a transition from school to the work environment.

PROGRAM OBJECTIVE

A long range objective of the STP was for the participant to be accepted into a community sheltered workshop. A short term objective was for the participant to develop work-related behaviors and basic skills as a foundation upon which the facility staff can evaluate the potential for vocational preparation.

PROGRAM METHODOLOGY AND STRATEGIES

Presenting a written proposal to the facility's administrators was the initial step in the program development process. The proposal detailed the participant selection process, the program purpose, the physical and operational structure and specific examples of the work sample tasks. The compensation system, a token economy, was also described, as well as an intrafacility system for ongoing program operations. The occupational therapy consultant's role in the STP was also defined.

Participant Selection

The participants in the initial STP group were to be the five highest scoring individuals among the total group tested using an informal, criterion-references assessment (i.e., a test that is constructed to yield measurements that are directly related to specific tasks rather than to the performance of other individuals) (Gronlund, 1981). These five top-performing individuals would be the model group; once their work-related behaviors were established, others would be added to the group. The minimum criteria to be considered for the model group addressed the most basic competencies one would need to productively participate in a workshop setting.

Basic Competencies Required for Participation

Basic competencies related to one's physical, perceptual and cognitive abilities provided the basis on which residents were selected to participate in the STP. The physical ability to reach, grasp and transfer objects was considered essential because the STP activities would involve manipulative tasks. Because several of the potential candidates for the program had varying degrees of visual impairment, visual abilities adequate to allow for gross discrimination between objects was an important consideration in the participant selection process. The capability to follow simple verbal commands such as "sit . . . wait . . . stop . . . raise your hand," as well as the ability to respond appropriately to "yes" and "no" was deemed an important ability for behavior management in the workshop setting. The last criterion (i.e., the arbitrarily selected duration of each work session) pertained to the tolerance and physical ability to remain seated for 15 minutes at a time between break periods. This criterion would limit the number of those residents who demonstrated frequent, uncontrolled grand mal seizures and those who experienced skin breakdown problems from qualifying for the STP by crediting them with lower points in this final category.

Participant Selection Evaluation

All candidates for the STP were to be assessed by the Resident Pre-Vocational Program Selection Evaluation prior to being placed in the program. The participants were then selected based on the performance scores.

Each of the four exercises of the Resident Pre-Vocational Program Selection Evaluation correlated with the minimum criteria described in the previous section. Exercise I focused primarily on the manipulative abilities, although one's ability to follow simple and complex directions and to apply simple perceptual concepts was also evaluated. For example, each candidate was instructed to pick up a block with one hand, transfer it to the opposite hand and replace the object on the table. Instructions were repeated with index cards and pencils replacing the block; the variety of objects grasped provided information on one's adaptive ability to handle various shaped objects.

Exercise II assessed functional eye-hand skills related to gross visual acuity. Specifically, it tested one's ability to accurately reach for and grasp varying sized objects. Exercise III, Receptive Language, related to one's ability to respond to one word commands (e.g., stop, faster, slower, wait, stand up) that would be used for basic behavior management in this program. Exercise IV, the last section, addressed one's physical ability to sit for 15 minutes by noting whether the individual could sit for 15 minutes in the absence of seizures or the threat of skin breakdown.

Scoring

A simple scoring system was used which required a minimum of staff time to score and interpret the results. Items were scored on a zero to two point scale; a stopwatch was used to record the time required by candidates to complete each item.

Staff

Two staff persons, the educator and speech pathologist, were to administer the Resident Pre-Vocational Participant Selection Evaluation and implement the STP. These full time staff were trained by the consultant to conduct the evaluation since they worked directly with those residents and would have some input regarding the ultimate selection of the first group of participants.

Training Program

The prospective residents in this new program had Individual Educational Plans (IEPs) or Individual Habilitation Plans (IHPs) involving motor programs, social habilitation and language programs. Developing work samples which would correlate with each of the IEPs and IHPs long range goals was the next area of concern.

Work Samples

Work Samples are simulated tasks or work activities for which there exists no industrial, business or other counterpart. Work samples are contrasted with *job samples*, which are models or reproduc-

Manipulative Ability

Accuracy Score Criteria

Points	Task Performance
2	Can do independently
1	Requires physical assistance and/or verbal prompting to complete
0	Cannot do (physically or cognitively incapable)

Materials Needed

Table & Chair (in a non-distracting room)
Stop Watch
10 - 1" cubes (2 each of red, green, yellow, blue and white)
10 - 3" x 5" Index cards
10 - pencils

Exercise I

A. Instruct student to pick up one (1) cube with one hand, transfer to opposite hand and place cube on table. Repeat instructions for all 10 cubes.

Score: _____
Time: _____
Comments: _____

FIGURE 1. Score system used to determine STP participant selection.

tions of a job that exist in an industrial, business or other setting. The STP only utilized work samples (Brolin, 1976).

The Stamping Activity in Figure 2 demonstrates how a work sample may incorporate progressive skill levels of performance.

Daily Operation

The STP was to be held in the same room daily, initially for one hour. This required the facility to provide a designated work space in which to house the program. The long range plan was to increase the scheduled time to one full morning several days per week. Each resident would be assigned to a work station to which he/she would be expected to return daily and after breaks. The plan also required that the facility provide a table or some type of work surface.

A punch card system using envelopes with the resident's name on each envelope would be stationed outside the workshop door. This system was designed to represent time cards to document attendance and punctuality. Prior to entering the work area, the staff person would punch the date and time that the resident entered. A clock, or a kitchen timer, was needed in the working arca to designate breaks and work periods.

The program had work and rest (break) periods at regularly scheduled intervals. A clock in the work area would have red and green dots on designated numbers to indicate "break" times and times when to return to work. The alarm clock or kitchen timer would alert the clients to the time intervals.

During work periods the participants' behaviors were to be monitored in terms of "on task behaviors" only. In this particular setting, the main behaviors observed were "no talking to others," "no touching others," and "attendance to the work sample."

The initial work samples were based on the participant's individual IEP/IHPs. The consultant personally trained each participant on the first work sample so that when the group met for the first time, the work periods could begin immediately, without time for training during the "workshop session."

Token System of Compensation

The plan was to develop a system of compensation for the participants whereby a token economy would be established. Initially,

STAMPING ACTIVITY

	TASK	MATERIALS	CRITERIA
1.	Stamp each paper on upper half of paper.	Rubber stamp; ink pad; paper all same color.	Stamp must be on upper half of paper; all papers must be stamped with only one stamp on each.
2.	Stamp each paper with a stamp designated for the paper color.	Two different rubber stamps; two colors of paper.	Each paper must be stamped one time in any position with the correct stamp for each color of paper.
3.	Same as "Level 2" except use three colors of paper. One sheet is to be left blank.	Two different rubber stamps; three colors of paper.	Paper will be correctly stamped. One sheet will be left blank.

FIGURE 2. Example of a work sample.

credit in the form of stars on a card would be earned merely for one's attendance. Later, work production rate (i.e., number of tasks correctly completed within a specified time) would be the basis for compensation. Each participant's performance would be rated against his/her past established performance. "Raises" would be earned when the individual's production rate increased by two percent or some arbitrary percentage representing progress. Figure 3 shows a data sheet was developed to document daily productivity rates.

Economic and Time Costs

The economic and time costs of the STP to the facility are described as follows. The primary cost of the program was the allocation of a room in which to implement the STP, a table on which to work, and two staff members to supervise it. Other costs included storage space in which to house the work samples; an alarm clock or kitchen timer for signaling work and break periods; and a notebook or file system for organizing the participants' Performance Data/ Productivity Sheets and Individual Educations Plans to which the work samples relate. A set of work samples would be created by using a variety of on-site materials and manipulative objectives from the occupational therapy department.

Methods by which to continually upgrade the work samples, to correlate the work samples with the participant's developmental areas of strength, to document the quality of the participant's work adjustment, and to remunerate the participants via a token economy would be developed prior to beginning the program.

PROGRAM CRITIQUE/RESULTS

The major obstacle to beginning the STP was finding a room in which to house the STP. There were no extra rooms so a large bedroom was used. This meant that materials and equipment had to be stored elsewhere, transported and set up each time the program was scheduled. Other staff were indirectly involved in the program. For example, Room Aides were responsible for getting the partici-

GROUP PROGRAM DOCUMENTATION SHEET
(Motor-Language-Social Habilitation Program)

Client's Name _Katrina_

Page Number _1_

Job# 1 _Color Sort- 2 colors_

Job# 2 _____

Job# 3 _____

Date	Production Rate Pcs. completed Total no. given X 100 = __	Materials	Observations/ Comments
4-8-88 # 1	$\frac{50 : 20}{40\,\%}$ per _20_ min. (min. = duration to complete the work sample)	25 blue blocks 25 red blocks	used ⓇR hand Placed one at a time Appeared unsure of matching colors Asked for assistance most of time.
4-8-88 # 1	$\frac{50 : 36}{70\,\%}$ per _20_ min.	Same	Needed much reinforcement & cueing most correct items in this job were corrected or cued
4-10-88 # 1	$\frac{50 : 47}{98\,\%}$ per _8_ min.	Same	Sorted all blue blocks first, then red appeared to be sorting by shade, not color Appeared to have muscle spasm in Ⓛ arm -nurse adm'd Tylenol - Katrina returned to class
4-15-88	$\frac{50 : 0}{0\,\%}$ per _8_ min.	25 blue blocks 25 red blocks	Placed all objects in one section.

FIGURE 3. Example of a completed work sample data sheet.

pants physically ready so that they could attend on time. House-keeping staff had to alter cleaning and floor waxing schedules. The wheelchair washing schedules had to be changed so that the STP participants' chairs were dry and available for use at the program's scheduled time.

The participants were extremely enthusiastic about attending the STP. After the consultant "interviewed" one participant to train her on the initial work sample, she returned to her room and triumphantly announced to the Room Aides, "They hired me. I got the job!"

The first set of staff in charge of the STP were the Special Educator and the Speech and Language Pathologist. The program was scheduled to meet twice/weekly, for one hour each session. This was in contrast to the suggested one hour per day schedule. Four 10 minute work sessions alternated with three five minute break periods, and the last five minutes was reserved for "clean up." The program seemed to run smoothly for three months, both from staff reports and the consultant's observations.

In the fourth month of operation there were set-backs in the form of staff turnover, a common occurrence in a residential facility. The Special Educator and the Speech and Language Pathologist resigned. The STP was "on hold" for about seven weeks while new staff were being assigned to the program by the administration.

The consultant provided inservice training to the new staff in the same manner as the first group but due to the educational differences between the new staff and that of the first group, numerous complaints about the feasibility of the program soon began to surface. The most prevalent complaints were (1) the data sheet was too complicated to use; (2) it was too difficult to get all of the participants to work at one time; and (3) more help was needed as there was too much to do for two staff persons. Other complaints related to the Room Aides, who failed to get the participants ready on time, and the exterminators and floor waxers from housekeeping, who chose to do their jobs during the time reserved for the STP and in the program's designated room.

After several months of sporadic operations the consultant requested a meeting with the staff and supervisory personnel involved with the therapy programming to discuss and resolve the obstacles that seemed to continually occur. As a result of this meeting, the Special Educator, whose students attended the STP, replaced one of the staff previously assigned to the program. A method for controlling the interferences by housekeeping staff was devised, and the staff directly assigned to the STP were allowed to clear up misunderstandings regarding the work sample data sheets. In retrospect, this meeting should have occurred long before these problems became so pronounced and debilitating to the STP.

After one year of operation, the STP still appears to be functioning at its initial level. The token economy is just being implemented, although the participants have not experienced the challenges of a work program. Work samples have just recently been upgraded. The suggested half-day schedule for the program has not yet occurred, and with the present two hours per week that the participants do spend in the STP, it would be unrealistic to use this session to evaluate their work adjustment abilities.

The advantages of the program still outweigh the disadvantages. Although it is difficult for the staff at times, the administration is supportive of the program and the participants definitely look forward to attending it.

The benefit of developing work adjustment experiences within the facility is great. The advantages of the STP are that 1) the residents are more motivated to participate in the tasks presented in a work-related atmosphere than they were when similar activities were presented in an individual therapy setting; 2) the work adjustment experiences that the program offers each participant can only be developed in such a group setting; and 3) the participants are all developing a sense of reality orientation with respect to the time of the day and the days of the week. They eagerly look forward to 11:00 A.M. on Tuesdays and Thursdays and question the staff if there appears to be a disruption in their scheduled program.

The main disadvantage of the STP is the impact of the program on the ancillary staff (i.e., Room Aides and housekeeping staff), on staff involved with the resident just prior to the resident's preparation for attending the program, and on those who have duties related to the maintenance of the room in which the program occurs.

Staff have noticed definite academic and social maturity gains within the individual STP participants. One resident's frequent inappropriate outbursts have decreased markedly because he is allowed to attend or remain in the program *only* if he is socially appropriate. Another resident has developed functional use of numerical concepts which he is able to apply outside of the STP. A sense of competition to excel and achieve is also developing between two brothers who are both in the program.

In retrospect, establishing definite time lines for initiating various phases of the program might have been helpful. Also, having a staff overlap between "new" and "departing" staff might have eliminated some of the detailed inservice training that had to be repeated. However, the problem of staff turnover is the single most threatening element to the smooth flow of such a program, and the luxury of having staff overlap may not always be possible.

In addition to the obstacles to the STP as detailed above, the occupational therapy consultant's inability to directly supervise the program during the first few sessions seemed to influence its smooth flow. The role of the occupational therapy consultant included other responsibilities to the facility beside the STP. Therefore, the four hours per week could not be spent exclusively on this project. When problems or questions arose regarding the STP, the staff had to wait until the following week to voice concerns and seek advice.

While the consultant can propose programs or make suggestions, she cannot directly implement either (Jaffe, 1988). In this situation, the occupational therapy consultant had no control over the selection of personnel selected to run the STP, although her suggestion to assign one of the COTA's to this program was accepted. She was unable to control the STP's daily schedule, therefore the administration scheduled it on a day other than her scheduled consultation day.

CONCLUSION

The key element in the success of such an endeavor as the STP appears to be dependent upon the staff who are directly involved with its implementation. This seems to be independent of the clarity with which the program is written or *who* is indirectly supervising it.

The consultant's ability to motivate the staff directly involved in the program is a key factor in their intrinsic commitment to the program. The occupational therapy consultant can serve as a resource for upgrading the work samples, designing new ones, and evaluating the participants' competencies in the program.

The STP addresses the pressing need, presented by Brolin

(1982), to realign the educational programs with the rehabilitation programs. Appropriate techniques need to be developed that will aid individuals with mental retardation in their transitions from the classroom to the community. Vocational preparation of the individual with developmental disabilities is an extremely complex process. However according to Brolin (1976, p. 65) ". . . Society places a high value on the activity of work, (so) let us give everyone the opportunity for achieving this important goal."

REFERENCES

Brolin, D. (1976). *Vocational preparation of retarded citizens*. Columbus, OH: Charles E. Merrill.

Brolin, D. (1982). *Vocational preparation of persons with handicaps* (2nd ed.). Columbus, OH: Charles E. Merrill.

Gronlund, N. (1981). *Measurement and evaluation in teaching* (4th ed.). New York: Macmillan Publishing Co., Inc.

Hopkins, H. & Smith, H. (1983). *Willard and Spackman's Occupational Therapy* (6th ed.). Philadelphia, PA: Lippincott Co.

Jaffe, E. (1988). The occupational therapist as a consultant: A model of community consultation. *Occupational Therapy in Health Care, 5* (1), 87-108.

Kielhofner, B., Burke, J., & Igi, C. (1980). A model of human occupation, Part 4. Assessment and intervention. *American Journal of Occupational Therapy, 34* (12), 777-788.

Reilly, M. (1962). Occupational therapy can be one of the great ideas of 20th century medicine. *American Journal of Occupational Therapy, 16* (1), 1-9.

Scott, M., Ebbert, A., & Price. D. (1986). Assessing and teaching employability skills with prevocational work samples. *The Directive Teacher, 8* (1), 3-5.

Stephens, T.M. (1978). *Social skills in the classroom*. Columbus, OH: Cedars Press, Inc.

Wehman, P., Kregel, J., & Barcus, J.M. (1985). From school to work: A vocational transition model for handicapped students. *Exceptional Children, 52* (1), 25-27.

Weisgerber, R., Dahl, P., & Appleby, J. (1981). *Training the handicapped for productive employment*. Rockville, MD: Aspen Systems Corp.

Developmental Growth in "ACTION": A Pilot Program for the Adult Retarded

Jane T. Herrick, OTR
Helen E. Lowe, OTR

SUMMARY. This paper describes a pilot program in a work activity center. Called the "ACTION Group," the project involved six clients whose selection was based on low productivity rates on work assignments. The purpose of the "ACTION Group" was to allow clients who were experiencing failure to be motivated by tasks structured to their performance needs. The hypothesis is that productivity improves when clients are presented with purposeful and appealing activities at their developmental level.

Sheltered workshops have been for many years a vocational setting for the adult retarded population. These facilities ideally provide assessment, training, and employment. Work activity centers were developed for those individuals with retardation who could benefit from a work-related program, but for various reasons were not appropriate for the more stringent demands of sheltered workshops. The research for this pilot project was done at the work activity levels.

BACKGROUND

The "ACTION" program was designed and implemented by occupational therapists at the New Opportunity Workshop, Inc., a work activity center in Pasadena, California. It was designed to

---

Jane T. Herrick and Helen E. Lowe are consultants in mental retardation and the authors of the Adult Skills Evaluation Survey for Persons with Mental Retardation (ASES). They are associated with the New Opportunity Workshops, Inc., 770 North Fair Oaks Avenue, Pasadena, CA 91103.

determine if vocationally unproductive clients would improve by participating in a structured program of activities appropriate to their developmental level. In the Information Packet on Mental Retardation by the American Occupational Therapy Association (Revised 1985), the concept is acknowledged that when activities are significantly related to the developmental interests of the individual, they offer the necessary learning for growth or restoration.

The New Opportunity Workshop trains 60 adult men and women who have a primary diagnosis of mild to moderate retardation. Specializing in packaging, assembling and mailing, the focus of vocational training is on sub-contract work for companies in the Southern California area. Vocational coordinators provide direct client supervision on the job. One function of the rehabilitation coordinator is to calculate client paychecks based on the Earned Industrial Standard Unit (EISU). The EISU is based on the standard number of units an able-bodied person can do in a 50 minute hour.

The "ACTION" group was conducted by two occupational therapists to investigate the concept that intensive, structured, developmentally-oriented training sessions would improve vocational potential. One criterion for inclusion in the target group was a production rate of ten percent or less on the EISU scale. The other requirement was a current vocational assessment score from the Adult Skills Evaluation Survey for Persons with Mental Retardation (ASES), (1985). This instrument, developed and published by the authors, established the level of client performance skills and was basic to refining the training methods used in this demonstration project.

PROGRAM

Six clients were chosen who met the criteria of a low production rate and a skills assessment score. A control group of six clients was identified who also rated ten percent or less on the EISU, and had similar scores on the ASES. These clients continued working on sub-contract jobs full-time, with no special intervention.

The weekly two-and-one-half-hour sessions focused on a variety of work-related activities. Based on the therapists' research and experience, they adapted items from the following assessments: Gesell Developmental Diagnosis (1974), Bayley Scales of Infant Development (1969), Vineland Social Maturity Scale (1965), Bruininks-Oseretsky Tests (1946), Memphis Instruments for Individual Program Planning and Evaluation (1974), and Watch Me Grow (1977).

The activities were selected from the five year and underdevelopmental levels at which the participants were functioning. The tasks were role appropriate and designed to be purposeful and appealing to the clients, motivating active participation, and promoting perception and improved performance. The activities stressed the sensory functions of attending, listening, and responding. The hypothesis was that productivity for clients experiencing failure improved when they were presented tasks structured at their identified performance levels.

The therapists conducted the developmental program in a setting that offered a minimum of distraction. The format was work-related and instruction was both verbal and visual. The specific activities chosen reflected the therapists' training in occupational therapy methods, experience with this population, and availability of materials within the training center. The order of task presentation followed a pattern which was repeated at each session to offer reinforcement. This simple repetitive format provided the opportunity to explore individual abilities and limitations as well as observe the client's methods of coping with competition, frustration, and failure. Performance of the "ACTION" participants on individual tasks was monitored by observation and recorded at each session. The numerical values of zero, one, and two were used to indicate the level of task competence.

The sessions were divided into the following five areas:

- *Matching* tasks trained in color, form, size discrimination, accuracy, and decision making. The tasks included using simple shapes, formboards, and puzzles; matching objects to pictures; and copying designs on paper.
- *Numbers* from one to five were used to develop numerical concepts. This activity included following directions such as counting a specific number of objects, tapping in rhythm, and counting aloud in numerical sequence.

- *Exercises* were designed to improve body image, increase endurance and postural awareness. One set, performed seated, involved the upper body with emphasis on hands, arms, shoulders and head. The other set, performed standing, used gross motor abilities such as bending, stretching, and balancing.
- *Language* activities centered around listening and responding. This required such non-verbal responses as pointing to objects and following 3-step sequences. Verbal responses included naming objects and body parts and answering questions.
- *Vocational* projects, with instruction that was both verbal and visual, addressed manual skills, quality of work, speed, and perseverance. The tasks used were folding, collating, sorting, and inspecting which represented various types of production jobs sub-contracted in a work activity center.

APPROACH

During this project, the therapists worked closely with the vocational coordinators and the rehabilitation coordinator. Scheduling staff members to observe clients functioning in this controlled learning environment enabled them to recognize individual competencies and potential for improvement in production. It also gave them opportunity to observe social interaction which could then be integrated into training strategies.

The clients selected for the "ACTION" group were experiencing chronic failure in their work setting with problems related to behavior and productivity. During the pilot program, they maintained a level of concentration satisfactory for performance on work-related jobs. This observation supports the need to present a variety of tasks to low functioning clients in a structured program in order to achieve success in vocational goals.

A program of this type should advance understanding of the obstacles that affect the behavior, reasoning, and coping mechanisms of adults with retardation under work-related conditions. Gary Kielhofner has aptly stated,

One of the most severely limiting features in the life of the severely disabled is the inability or unwillingness of others to recognize or grant competence to their efforts and performance because they differ from the average. What would be a good performance for a person with a radically altered brain or body? The answer to the question lies both in the perspective (however limited or deviant) of the individual and the ability of another to recognize and appreciate performance from the same perspective. (Kielhofner, 1983, p.262)

RESULTS

At the conclusion of this pilot project, the difference between production rates of the "ACTION" and control groups was determined from the Earned Industrial Standard Unit records. These data were used to test the statistical significance through the use of a t test. The t value was 2.85 which was significant at the +.05 level. Figures from the EISU showed that three clients in the "ACTION" group made gains in production while three maintained their previous work level. In the control group, one client gained in productivity, two maintained the work level, and three lost percentage points.

DISCUSSION

The small number of participants and the short duration of the project dictate caution in interpreting results. However, a practice model such as the "ACTION" group serves to suggest the need for further research on functional performance of adults with retardation. This pilot project seems to indicate that work-related programming, structured at the client's level of achievement, can improve productivity and behavior. Although therapists working with persons with retardation must be satisfied with small gains and slow progress, they need to recognize that persons at all levels of retardation can learn (Schulman, 1980).

IMPLICATIONS FOR OCCUPATIONAL THERAPY

There have been for years forward-looking therapists such as Florence Cromwell who have advocated community-based settings for the profession. Unfortunately, the tendency of the occupational therapist to gravitate toward the more secure and lucrative Jobs in traditional and well established clinics and institutions often makes them unavailable to the population which needs them in a community setting (Morse, 1987).

In her presidential address in 1987, Elnora Gilfoyle challenged therapists to promote the potential resources of persons who are chronically disabled:

> Occupational therapy's philosophical grounding lies in its commitment to serve citizens with severe and chronic disabilities and perceive them as valued populations who have a right to human dignity and productive living. Our commitment is not popular because the persons we serve are frequently considered "devalued" populations in America's culture. Society's negative attitude toward chronic impairments is a challenge we must face in our efforts to assure occupational therapy's position in the marketplace. (Gilfoyle, 1987, p.779)

REFERENCES

American Occupational Therapy Association Inc., Division of Professional Development (1981). *Mental Retardation*, Rockville, MD: American Occupational Therapy Association.

American Occupational Therapy Foundation Inc., (1977). *Watch Me Grow*, Rockville, MD: American Occupational Therapy Foundation, Inc.

Bayley, N. (1969). *Bayley Scales of Infant Development*, New York: The Psychological Corporation.

Bruininks, R. (1978). *Bruininks-Oseretsky Test of Motor Proficiency*, Circle Pines, MN: American Guidance Service Inc.

Doll, E. (1965). *Vineland Social Maturity Scale*, Circle Pines, MN: American Guidance Service Inc.

Gesell, A. and Amatrada, C. (1974). *Developmental Diagnoses 2nd ed.* Maryland: Harper & Row.

Gilfoyle, E. (1987). Creative partnerships: The profession's plan, *American Journal of Occupational Therapy* 41, 779-781.

Herrick, J. and Lowe, H. (1985). *The Adult Skills Evaluation Survey for Persons with Mental Retardation*, Pasadena, CA: Published by the authors.

Kielhofner, G. (1983). *Health Through Occupation*, Philadelphia, PA: F.A. Davis.

Memphis State University (1974). *Project Memphis Instruments for Individual Program Planning and Evaluation*, Belmont, CA: Lear Siegler, Inc./Fearon.

Morse, A. (1987). A cultural intervention model for developmentally disabled adults: An expanded role for occupational therapists, *Occupational Therapy in Health Care*, 4, 103-113.

Schulman, E. (1980), *Focus on the Retarded Adult*, St. Louis, MO: C.V. Mosby Co.

Options:
An Occupational Therapy Transition Program for Adolescents with Developmental Disabilities

Jeanne Jackson, MA, OTR
Allyn Rankin, OTR
Sue Siefken, MA, OTR
Florence Clark, PhD, OTR, FAOTA

SUMMARY. This article discusses a grant-funded occupational therapy independent living skills transition program for adolescents with developmental disabilities on a non-mainstreamed high school campus. The Options Program was designed to provide intensive transition services through its emphasis on exploring and broadening the range of individuals' choices' about employment, living arrangements, and social activities. The assessment procedure, program model, curriculum goals, and intervention strategies are presented.

Jeanne Jackson is Adjunct Instructor, Department of Occupational Therapy, University of Southern California; and Options Program Director, Hope Special Education Center. Allyn Rankin is an Options Program Preceptor, Hope Special Education Center. Sue Siefken is an Options Program Preceptor, Hope Special Education Center. Florence Clark is Associate Professor and Chair, Department of Occupational Therapy, University of Southern California; and Project Director of the OSERS Grant #G 008715563.

The authors wish to gratefully acknowledge Judy Dona-Bauer, Agnes Harai, Vickie Pennington, Shelly Sutfin, and Linda Watson, for their contributions to the original writing of the Options grant. Carolyn Snyder, deserves recognition for her contribution to the ideas expressed in this article.

INTRODUCTION

"The transition from school to working life calls for a range of choices about career options, living arrangements, social life and economic goals that often have lifelong consequences" (Will, 1985, p. 1). In this quote, Madeline Will, the Assistant Secretary of the Office of Special Education and Rehabilitative Services (OSERS), acknowledges the comprehensive nature of the transition from the role of adolescence to that of adult life.

For high school students with disabilities, the successful transition from a structured and protected school environment to an unstructured community environment is often an overwhelming task (Pennington & Sharrott, 1985). Their task is further complicated by a paucity of transition services at both the high school and community levels. As a result, students' desires and efforts to prepare themselves to assume the adult role and be productive members of society are stifled. Modifying the approach toward educating students with disabilities and expanding the transition services offered at the high school and community levels are needed.

In 1984, OSERS responded to these needs by establishing "transition" as the decade's priority of special education (Wills, 1985). This national policy set aside funding to develop high school transition programs, to train professionals to become transition experts, and to generate research on the efficacy of transition programming. Dr. Florence Clark at the University of Southern California Department of Occupational Therapy has received two grants from OSERS and has been extensively involved in the design and implementation of transition services for the last 5 years. Initially, funding was awarded to establish an Independent Living Skills Transition Center on a mainstreamed high school campus for students with emotional, communication, learning, and multiple disabilities. A more recent grant enabled an extension of these services to include transition programming for adolescents with developmental disabilities attending the Hope Special Education Center (Hope), a non-mainstreamed high school campus located in Buena Park, California.

The purpose of this article is to describe the Options Program, an occupational therapy transition program for high school students with developmental disabilities. First, the frame of reference guiding the design of the program will be presented. Second, the Options Program, including assessment procedures, curriculum goals, and the parent component will be described.

FRAME OF REFERENCE

The development of the Options Program at the Hope School was heavily influenced by the philosophical tenets of the Independent Living Movement (ILM), a grass-roots socio-political movement which emerged during the late 1960s and early 1970s. The intent of this movement was to reshape society's view of disability from one in which the person with a disability is perceived as a charity case to one in which the individual is seen as a productive, responsible member of society, deserving of the same rights as those without disability (DeJong, 1983).

The founders of the ILM planned to accomplish this task by effecting a change in service provision, research direction, and legislation for persons with disabilities (DeJong, 1983). The ILM proposed a new perspective on disability which expands opportunities for persons with disabilities to participate in quality life experiences. Four distinguishing concepts associated with this new perspective will be presented to illustrate our approach toward the students we serve through the Options Program.

The proponents of the ILM viewed independence as a mind process (Cole, 1983; DeJong, 1983; Zola, 1983). Rather than focusing on the number of "mundane tasks" a person can complete without assistance, advocates argued that self-direction is the critical factor which separates disability from independence (DeJong & Wenker, 1983; Varela, 1983; Zola, 1983). They strongly asserted that people with disabilities have the right to control their own lives and that self-direction, participation in day-to-day decision making, is of equal importance to task completion. The proponents claimed that, in traditional rehabilitation services, greater emphasis is placed on the individual's performance of an activity without assistance and lesser emphasis is placed on fostering self-direction (DeJong & Wenker, 1983; Varela, 1983). For persons with developmental disabilities, this is a vital concern.

Studies have shown that one's ability to use proper judgment, interact effectively with others, and problem solve is often a determining factor in whether one will meet with success or failure within the work setting (Mithaug, Martin, & Agran, 1987). The results of these studies point to the importance of accepting the broad view of independence endorsed by the ILM.

When this philosophical shift in the view of independence is applied to practice, one can see remarkable opportunities for different approaches and priorities in developing treatment goals. Cultivating a student's ability for self-direction, autonomy, decision making, and problem solving becomes of tantamount importance.

Advocates of the ILM do not exclude skill acquisition as a treatment goal, but rather dictate that the process through which one learns new skills must always present opportunities for self-direction and solving problems (Cole, 1987). For example, when programs to promote employment upon graduation are designed, environments must be created which include an element of choice, present challenges, and demand spontaneous decision making and use of judgment. In addition, ample opportunity to develop and practice task-specific skills which meet the expectations of the employer must be allowed.

Consistent with this view of independence, students in the Options Program are active participants in their programming, thus fostering the development of self-direction (Cole, 1983). The students are expected to assist in establishing their individual programs by expressing their preferences for job placements, leisure activities, and possible future living situations. Opportunities for skill development are presented in areas which the student identifies as needed.

A second critical concept of the ILM paradigm is the individual's need for and right to engage in risk-taking behaviors. DeJong (1983) stated: "The dignity of risk is at the heart of the Independent Living Movement. Without the possibility of failure, the disabled person lacks true independence, the ultimate mark of humanity, the right to choose" (p. 20). This statement clearly captures the message that individuals have a drive for engaging in behaviors that create a sense of challenge and involve an element of risk.

Through experimentation with alternative responses to daily

problems and experiencing the consequences of their choices, individuals build the resources and problem-solving skills needed to contend with the future complexities of adult roles. Challenges and risks for persons with developmental disabilities are often inherent in the unpredictability and uncertainty of everyday events (Perske, 1972). Despite the need for including risk in their lives, persons with disabilities are often protected from or denied participation in these daily challenges (Cole, 1983; Gliedman & Roth, 1980). The ILM rejects this protection, stating that persons with disabilities have the right to confront and conquer the challenge and dilemmas associated with everyday experiences.

If adolescents are to assume adult roles, these opportunities to experience success or failure must be readily accessible and encouraged. The Options Program focuses on this need to provide nurturing, yet realistic, opportunities for students to experience the natural consequences of their choices in a variety of work and community settings. Careful attention is given to encouraging risk-taking behaviors and participation in challenges presented by daily life situations despite the fact that the challenges may appear too complex and overwhelming for the student.

The third concept which warrants discussion involves the rights of persons with disabilities to assume the variety of roles enjoyed by the non-disabled adult population which may include the roles of family member, worker, volunteer, and social participant. Many of these roles are, simply, unattainable for persons with disabilities.

The values and beliefs underlying the medical model contribute to the prohibition of persons with disabilities from engaging in the complete spectrum of adult roles. Influenced by the values of the medical model, society confines persons with disabilities to either the sick or impaired role (Yerxa, 1983). Societal expectations that the "sick/disabled" individual should be relieved from familial, occupational, and civic responsibilities are inherent in the sick or impaired role. Proponents of the ILM acknowledge these expectations as unjust, claiming that adults with disabilities do not wish to be deprived of the joys and responsibilities associated with adult roles (DeJong, 1983).

On the contrary, persons with disabilities seek the opportunity to become equipped with the skills needed to participate successfully as a family member, employee, volunteer, and social participant. It is only when persons with disabilities possess the skills and behavior inherent in adult roles that they are free to choose alternatives in life. The Options Program addresses this concern raised by the ILM by facilitating the development of skills and behaviors associated with a variety of adult roles. Three areas of adult life are emphasized: residence in the least restrictive environment, employment, and participation in a social/leisure network (Halpern, 1985).

Finally, if a transition program to further the independence of students is to be developed, one must ask, "What are the various factors which impede the individual's achievement of independence?" The ILM philosophy places heavy blame on the rehabilitation process, social attitudes, political controls, and architectural barriers as the major impediments to successful community integration for persons with disabilities (Varela, 1983).

Attitudes of parents, teachers, and rehabilitation professionals can shape an individual's perception of his or her abilities (Cole, 1983). A home or school environment in which an absence of challenges exists will encourage individuals to remain passive recipients of life rather than active participants. Proponents of the ILM believe that this is the case in traditional rehabilitation and that these aspects of the rehabilitation process impede the acquisition of independence (Cole, 1983; DeJong, 1983; Zola, 1983).

Social barriers toward independence can occur, for example, when the stigma associated with requiring special considerations may bar an employer from first hiring someone with a disability. Political barriers are present in the laws which create work disincentives for persons with disabilities. Finally, architectural barriers can be found in the presence of stairs, as opposed to ramps, which can inhibit a person's access to a building.

Removing the barriers present in the work and community environments and in the political system is one of the goals of the Options Program. During the assessment phase, barriers to independence which exist within the students' environment are identified. Plans to change existing obstacles are incorporated into the student program. Changing the attitudes of employers, apartment managers, and the community in general is attempted through community contacts and by teaching parents to become effective advocates for their adolescents.

To summarize, the ILM emphasizes four themes specific to transition programming for adolescents with developmental disabilities. First, environments must be created which stimulate the development of self-direction skills. Second, opportunities to engage in risk-taking behaviors should be provided. Third, the development of skills consistent with adult life roles should be encouraged. Fourth, a concerted effort must be made to remove barriers which prevent independence.

THE OPTIONS PROGRAM

The Options Program was designed to address the need for more extensive transition services for high school students with developmental disabilities. The program, in existence since September, 1988, serves 20 of the 110 students with developmental disabilities who attend this non-mainstreamed school. The Hope School's curriculum offers the students independent living training and opportunities for campus and community-based work experiences. The Options Program is designed to complement these existing services and to enhance the students' transition to adult roles.

Figure 1 illustrates the transition process from the Hope School to adult community life. One pillar of the bridge depicts the activities which comprise the student role. The other pillar represents the activities that students must be prepared to fulfill as adults: employment, independent living, and effective social interaction.

The Hope School's independent living curriculum and vocational experiences and the Options Program help construct the bridge that spans the transition from school to community life. The Options Program contributes to the Hope School curriculum by providing more intensive transition services through its emphasis on exploring and broadening the range of one's choices about employment, living arrangements, and social activities, and creating opportunities for individuals to gain a variety of experiences in these areas. The assessment procedure, curriculum, and parent involvement will be described.

204

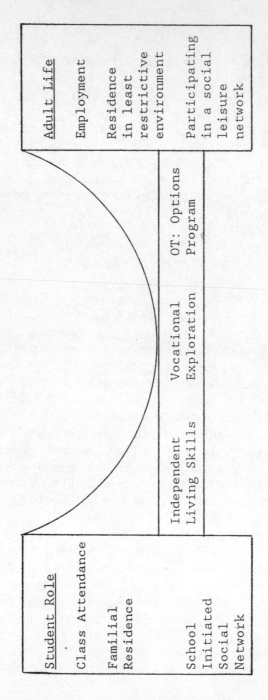

FIGURE 1

ASSESSMENT

The first stage of the Options Program consists of an extensive evaluation of the students' transition needs. Six assessments were selected or designed to elicit information in four domains: 1) task-specific skills and interests in the area of independent living, work, and leisure activities; 2) self-concept; 3) future aspirations; and 4) self-direction skills. (For the purpose of these evaluations, self-direction skills include risk taking, flexibility, persistence, self-initiation, constancy of behavior, decision making, problem solving, judgment, and social interaction skills (Cole, 1983).) Student assessments include a naturalistic observation, the *Interest Checklist* (Matsutsuyu, 1969), the *Cantril Ladder* (Cantril, 1965), the *Piers-Harris Self-Concept Scale* (Piers, 1985), and a Student Needs Assessment. Parents' perceptions and needs are evaluated through a Parent Needs Assessment. A combination of a naturalistic qualitative approach and the traditional quantitative approach was employed in the assessment procedure. Each evaluation used will be described.

Student Assessments

Naturalistic Observation

The naturalistic approach toward evaluation was chosen to identify the self-direction skills of the student which are difficult to ascertain through more traditional measurements such as questionnaires and checklists (Cole, 1983; Guba, 1986). Skills such as risk taking, persistence, problem solving, and self-initiation fall into this domain. For the Options Program, the naturalistic assessment constitutes a significant part of the evaluation procedure and provides information in the domains of self-direction skills and task-specific skills and interests.

Descriptive data are obtained through direct observation of students in three natural settings: home, work or school, and the community. Observing students in a variety of environments with varying elements of familiarity, novelty, structure, and flexibility provides insight into the students' repertoires of behaviors and skills which will be needed for living successfully in the community.

To initiate the observation, the therapist arrives at the student's home in the morning before the student departs for school or work. The home setting allows the therapist to observe the students in a familiar, routine environment. Interactions between the students, siblings, and parents as well as family attitudes about the student's capabilities are a primary focus for observation in this setting. Students are then followed to their work experience site, which represents a more structured environment. Task-specific skills, ability for self-direction, and adherence to rules established by the employer are observed. Finally, students are observed in an unfamiliar community situation, for example, a store or leisure activity. Again, the focus of the observation is the student's ability for self-direction. Following the observation, an interview with the student is completed to provide insights as to his or her own phenomenological experience in each setting. From the observation, a picture of the student's skills and behaviors in a variety of settings, important to a successful transition to adult roles upon graduation, is formulated.

Quantitative Evaluation

Several quantitative evaluations were selected or designed to assess students in the four domains mentioned above. The following paragraphs describe these evaluations.

Piers-Harris Children's Self-Concept Scale (Piers, 1985). This is a self-report inventory which measures self-concept in six categories. Students are requested to answer "Yes" or "No" to a variety of descriptive statements designed to tap their self-perception in the areas of intellect and school status, physical appearance, attribution of anxiety, popularity, happiness, and satisfaction.

Interest Checklist (Matsutsuyu, 1969). The *Interest Checklist* is an inventory on which students are asked to rate their interest in 80 activities as casual, strong, or none.

Cantril Ladder (Cantril, 1965). The *Cantril Ladder* measures overall life satisfaction. On a nine-step ladder, students are asked to indicate where they perceive themselves in relation to the "best possible life" or "worst possible life." The students' perceived life satisfaction is assessed in the present, 5 years prior, and 5 years into the future.

Student Needs Assessments. This questionnaire requires the respondent to identify independent living needs in the areas of residence, employment, and social activities. Information on specific task performance in each of these areas and future goals is requested.

Parent Assessment

Parent Needs Assessment. This questionnaire asks parents to rate the degree of independence their adolescents' have achieved in specific daily living tasks and self-direction skills such as decision making and self-initiation. The assessment also asks parents to describe the student's present living situation, plans for a future living situation, and which community agencies, if any, the student currently uses. Parents' needs with regard to their adolescents are solicited.

THE CURRICULUM

The Options Program, which was implemented in September, 1988, is pictured in Figure 2. The program spans a 4-semester or 2-year time period in which four curriculum themes are covered: independent living exploration, employment exploration, supported work experience, and community linkages. Students progress from the first year, where they focus on exploring options, to the second year where they gain practical experience. Each semester will be highlighted emphasizing the objectives and intervention strategies.

Semester One focuses on independent living exploration. Two primary objectives have been specified. The first objective is to introduce students to the concept of living in the least restrictive environment and to assist them in exploring their options in this area. The assumption is not made that every student will move to an independent living setting upon graduation. The intent of this objective is to expose the students to a variety of living situations so that students and parents will be aware of their choices and will know what existing community services can assist them in reaching short

	YEAR ONE		YEAR TWO	
	Semester One	Semester Two	Semester Three	Semester Four
ASSESSMENT	Independent Living Exploration	Employment Exploration	Supported Work	Supported Work
GRADUATION				Community Linkages

FIGURE 2

208

and long-term residential goals. Visits to a variety of settings (residential independent living training centers, homes of adults with disabilities, and cooperative living situations) will assist students to envision themselves living independently. In addition, adults with disabilities will serve as important role models by sharing with the students the benefits and challenges they encounter in their particular living situations. Students will be encouraged to identify their own preferences for independent living through follow-up discussion and activities.

Participating in a social leisure network of friends and actively contributing to the community by taking part in civic responsibilities are important to the enactment of adult roles and one's self-esteem. Therefore, the second objective is to provide students the opportunity to explore their options for leisure activities and expose them to the concept of community involvement. Initially, students will take responsibility for selecting a variety of social activities in which they wish to engage. As their interests in particular leisure activities emerge, the students will assist in planning a group or individual event in their respective areas of interest. Finally, each student will develop a week-end leisure schedule and plan the steps needed to carry out his or her week-end activities successfully.

Community involvement is addressed by introducing the concept of volunteerism. Volunteer experiences offer students the opportunity to fulfill the helper role associated with adulthood rather than their usual "helped" role associated with their childhood. As a group, students will be expected to choose one community event for which they wish to volunteer their time. The therapist will organize the volunteer experience with the agency and structure the tasks which are required of the students.

Semester Two: Employment Exploration. The second semester is designed to facilitate students' exploration of various employment options and job training agencies. Typically, students' work experiences depend on the availability of work sites rather than student interest. As part of the Options Program, students are encouraged to identify jobs in which they are the most interested and which they perceive as matching their personal attributes. Students can visit a variety of entry-level positions which may include clerical assistant, animal care assistant, beautician's aide, and grocer's assistant, as well as other job sites individually requested by the student. This process will lay the groundwork for the third semester, during which work experience sites based on each student's stated preferences are established.

The second objective for semester two is to introduce students to job placement and training agencies. As students are exposed to an array of vocational paths, they are able to form more realistic goals. Often, their goals crystallize around the time of graduation or after graduation. Students need to be aware of state or community agencies which offer job training and placement services for persons with disabilities. Strategies to accomplish this objective include inviting guest speakers from community agencies to discuss their services with students and parents, and visiting adults with disabilities at their supported job sites to discuss the process through which they attained their jobs.

Semester Three. Exploration experiences of the first and second semesters culminate in the second year of the Options Program as students prepare for graduation. The objective of the third semester is to enable the students to gain work experience at selected job sites based on their interests and preferences identified in semester two. Students will select a minimum of two non-traditional job experiences in which they will participate for two semesters. The therapist will be responsible for establishing contacts with employers and providing students with job experiences consistent with their interests. While some judgment on the part of the therapist will be utilized in placing the students in the jobs of their choice, every attempt will be made to allow the students to select their work experience sites.

Following the model of supported employment, students initially will be trained by therapists at the work sites to perform job-specific tasks. After students are secure in their positions, assistance will be decreased gradually, allowing students to independently solve problems which arise, make spontaneous decisions, and experience the natural consequences of their actions (Cole, 1983). Work experiences will be structured to encourage risk-taking behaviors on the part of the students. If failure occurs, the role of the therapist will be to guide and support the student in re-evaluating the student's skills, behaviors, and goals, and to modify skills or choose a more appropriate placement.

During this semester, therapists will assume an advocate's role by working with potential employers to modify their attitudes toward hiring persons with disabilities and expanding job opportunities beyond traditional sites. Employers who are experienced in hiring persons with developmental disabilities and who perceive a goodness-of-fit between the individual and job tasks are more apt to request additional students. It is the intention of the program to encourage new employers to begin the same process.

Semester Four: Community Linkages. The final semester prior to graduation is devoted to establishing linkages with appropriate community agencies which will provide services upon graduation. Kailes and Weil (1985) stated that many persons with disabilities are often unable to act as their own case managers because they lack information about community resources. This concern is felt acutely by parents who question how their adolescents' needs will be met when they can no longer benefit from the high school services and must contend with complex community systems. To address these concerns, therapists will assist students and parents to strengthen community linkages which have been made through the 2 years. Representatives from appropriate community services will be requested to attend the student's final Individualized Educational Plans (IEP) meeting in order to facilitate the transfer of responsibilities from the high school to adult community service agencies. Assistance will be provided with the agencies' application process. Finally, students will graduate with a personal resource book listing contacts which have been established with community agencies in the areas of employment, independent living, and leisure.

A second strategy to facilitate the transition process will be to establish a coalition of potential adult community service providers for the student population in the Options Program. The purpose of the coalition will be twofold. First, these providers will serve as a resource for the student in developing his or her own plans following graduation. Students will be given the opportunity to meet the coalition members in groups and individually to discuss their options. Second, the coalition will provide an avenue for networking between the school and the community. Regular meetings will be held which are both educational and interactive. The process of problem solving in regard to different transition issues and identifying unaddressed concerns will be a primary focus of the meetings.

Parent Group

Parent/caregiver support is of key importance in attaining the students' plans and goals. Parents and caregivers are the student's most consistent advocates. As the students approach graduation and adulthood, transition can be seen by parents as "the great unknown." The transition process is complicated by a lack of information, the number of choices that must be made, the changing role of the student, and, most importantly, issues of dependence versus independence in these emerging adults. For this reason, a parent component was incorporated into the Options Program, offering education, consultation, and a support network. Through individual and group meetings, parents will be able to discuss the many issues they will encounter as their sons or daughters make the transition into adult community life. Opportunity to receive information, to ask questions, and to meet community service providers aid parents in coping with the changes they will face in the future. This opportunity will help to improve parents' advocacy skills and decrease their fear of uncertainty.

CONCLUSION

Occupational therapy offers a unique and vital role in the provision of transition services to adolescents with disabilities. The Options Program was designed to complement the existing high school curriculum and is implemented on a non-mainstreamed high school campus for persons with developmental disabilities. Program design includes an assessment period, a direct student service component, the establishment of a coalition of community agencies, and a parent education component. The content of our intensive community-based curriculum is designed to foster job and independent living exploration and acquisition. The curriculum comprises four modules; students progress from exploring vocational and independent living options to gaining experience in supported work environments and to establishing linkages with community agencies. This progression will assist the students to make a smoother transition to adult community life.

REFERENCES

Cantril, H. (1965). *The pattern of human concern*. New Brunswick: Rutgers University Press.

Cole, J. A. (1983). Skills training. In N. Crewe & I. Zola (Eds.), *Independent living of physically disabled people*. San Francisco: Jossey-Bass.

DeJong, G. (1983). Defining and implementing the independent living concept. In N. Crewe & I. Zola (Eds.), *Independent living of physically disabled people*. San Francisco: Jossey-Bass.

DeJong, G., & Wenker, T. (1983). Attendant care. In N. Crewe & I. Zola (Eds.), *Independent living of physically disabled people*. San Francisco: Jossey-Bass.

Gliedman, J., & Roth, W. (1980). *The unexpected minority*. New York: Harcourt Brace Jovanovich.

Guba, E. G. (1986). What have we learned about naturalistic evaluation? Invitational Plenary Address, American Evaluation Association, Kansas City, MO, November 1, 1986.

Halpern, A. (1985). Transition: A look at the foundation. *Exceptional Children*, 5(6), 470-486.

Kailes, J. I., & Weil, M. (1985). People with disabilities and the independent living model. In M. Weil, J. M. Karls & Associates (Eds.), *Case management in human service practice*. San Francisco: Jossey-Bass Publishers.

Matsutsuyu, J. S. (1969). The interest checklist. *American Journal of Occupational Therapy*, 23, 323-328.

Mithaug, D. E., Martin, J. E., & Agran, M. (1987). Adaptability instruction: The goal of transitional programming. *Exceptional Children*, 53(6), 500-505.

Pennington, V., & Sharrott, G. W. (1985). The developmental tasks of adolescence and the role of occupational therapy. In F. S. Cromwell (Ed.), *Occupational therapy and adolescents with disability* (Vol. 2). New York: The Haworth Press.

Perske, R. (1972). The dignity of risk and the mentally retarded. *Mental Retardation*, 10.

Piers, E. (1985). *Piers-Harris children's self-concept scale, Revised manual*. Los Angeles: Western Psychological Services.

Varela, R. A. (1983). Changing social attitudes and legislation regarding disability. In N. Crewe & I. Zola (Eds.), *Independent living of physically disabled people*. San Francisco: Jossey-Bass.

Will, M. (1985). Transition: Linking disabled youth to a productive future. *OSERS News in Print*, *1*(1).

Yerxa, E. J. (1983). Audacious values. In G. Kielhofner (Ed.), *Health through occupation: Theory and practice in occupational therapy*. Philadelphia: F. A. Davis.

Zola, I. (1983). Toward independent living: Goals and dilemmas. In N. Crewe & I. Zola (Eds.), *Independent living of physically disabled people*. San Francisco: Jossey-Bass.

Grip Strength and Dexterity in Adults with Developmental Delays

Carol S. Transon, MOT, OTR
Christine K. Nitschke, BS, OTR
James J. McPherson, MS, OTR
Sandi J. Spaulding, MS, OTR
Gail A. Rukamp, OTR
Lisa M. Anderson, OTR
Patricia Hecht, OTR

SUMMARY. The purpose of this study was to determine the usefulness of dexterity and grip strength assessments by comparing the scores of adults with developmental delays with adult norms. A second purpose was to determine the correlations among the assessment instruments. Fifty-six developmentally disabled adults performed the box and block test, the nine hole peg test, and grip strength. Males performed significantly better on grip strength than females, but there was no significant difference on dexterity scores. Males scored significantly lower than established norms on all tests except the left nine hole peg test. Females scores were significantly lower than norms on all tests except the left and right nine hole peg test. Dexterity test scores on one side of the body were highly correlated

---

Carol S. Transon is affiliated with St. Coletta's School, W4955 Hwy 18, Jefferson, WI 53545. Christine K. Nitschke is affiliated with Evanston Hospital, 2650 Ridge Rd., Evanston, IL 60201. James J. McPherson and Sandi J. Spaulding are affiliated with the Program in Occupational Therapy, University of Wisconsin-Milwaukee, P.O. Box 413, Milwaukee, WI 53211. Gail A. Rukamp, Lisa M. Anderson, and Patricia Hecht are affiliated with the University of Wisconsin-Milwaukee.

The authors wish to thank the staff of St. Coletta's with special thanks to Sister E. Weber, Administrator, for their ongoing support for research, and to the subjects who kindly offered their time for this study.

Requests for reprints should be sent to: Carol S. Transon, Shared Therapeutic Services of Wisconsin, 3939 S. 92nd Street, Greenfield, WI 53228.

215

with those on the other side, but grip strength was not highly correlated with dexterity. This suggests that occupational therapists need to treat dexterity and grip as separate entities. The present results may provide guidelines to determine average performance for adults with developmental delays.

INTRODUCTION

Clinicians have observed that the adult developmentally disabled have performance deficits in tasks requiring dexterity and strength. However, no systematic study of these differences have been conducted among the adult developmentally delayed population. Recently, Mathiowetz et al., (1985a, 1985b, 1985c) have established adult norms for grip strength, gross manual dexterity and fine manipulative dexterity. The Jamar dynamometer was used to measure grip strength, the box and block test to measure gross manual dexterity, and the nine hole peg test to evaluate fine manipulative dexterity.

Mathiowetz et al., noted that although these tests were used extensively in clinics, a lack of standardized norms had compromised their use as valid assessment instruments. A test of these instruments with members of the adult mentally retarded population would provide clinicians with an estimate of their effectiveness as assessment tools for this population.

The primary purpose of this study was to determine the usefulness of these assessments by comparing scores of adult developmentally delayed individuals with presently available adult norms. A second purpose was to determine if there are correlations among the assessment instruments.

METHODOLOGY

Subjects

Fifty-six adults with developmental disabilities, between the ages of 21 and 66, volunteered as subjects. The mean age of this sample was 31. There were 28 males and 28 females. Intelligence scores ranged from 33 to 70 with a mean of 49.1. None of the subjects had any physical disabilities which could affect grip strength or dexterity. All subjects were enrolled in a residential facility, and each was his or her own guardian.

Procedures

The study took place in the occupational therapy clinic at St. Coletta's School, a familiar setting for the subjects. Three testing stations were set up in the room. The subjects rotated from one station to the next in an established order. At the first station the experimenter explained the purpose of the study, and the informed consent form was signed by the subject. At station number two another experimenter took strength measurements with a Jamar dynamometer and the nine hole peg test. The box and block test were administered at a third station by another experimenter. All testing was performed using standardized procedures as reported by Mathiowetz et al., (1985a, 1985b, 1985c). Testing took approximately half an hour for each subject.

Data Collection

Data were collected by registered occupational therapists and senior occupational therapy students who were trained in test administration.

The subjects carried a recording sheet which had their identifying code number. On the sheet there was a place for the examiner to record the results of each test. The subject performed each test three times and the mean of the three scores were used for analysis. The results of the nine hole peg test were recorded in number of seconds required to complete the task. The box and block test results were indicated by the number of blocks moved from one side of the box to the other in sixty seconds. The grip strength was measured in kilograms using the Jamar dynamometer. At the end of the test, the completed score sheet was given to the examiner at the first station in the testing room.

Data Analysis

Data for the male and female subjects were analyzed separately, then compared to norms established by Mathiowetz et al., (1985a, 1985b, 1985c). The Dunn-Bonferoni procedure (tD) was used to evaluate 18 planned contrasts (6 between male and female developmentally delayed subjects; 6 between developmentally delayed male subjects and established norms; and 6 between the female scores and the established norms). The two tailed critical value for tD is 18,28 (.95) = 3.28. Strength and dexterity results were correlated for each group using Pearson product moment correlation coefficients.

RESULTS

Male and Female Comparisons for the Developmentally Delayed Population

Male developmentally delayed individuals had significantly greater grip strength than females for both right and left hands (t = 5.48, t = 4.97 respectively). There were no noted differences between the two groups for gross dexterity using the box and block test and for fine manipulative dexterity using the nine hole peg tests (Table 1).

Developmentally Delayed Sample Compared to Established Norms

Both the male and female groups with developmentally delays scored significantly lower than the established norms for all tests, with the exception of the nine hole peg test for the left hand of males and both the left and the right hands of females (Table 2).

Correlations Among Grip Strength and Dexterity Variables

Left and right hand grip strength was highly correlated among both males and females. Grip strength and dexterity were correlated at low to moderate levels. Results using the nine hole peg test and the box and block test were more highly correlated among males than females. Correlations for males ranged from a high of − .7880 for the right hand box and block test/left hand nine hole peg test to a low of − .5961 for the right hand box and block/right hand nine hole peg). Correlations for females ranged from a high of − .6405

Table 1: Grip Strength and Dexterity Scores
of Subjects with Developmental Disabilities

Test	Males (N=28)		Females (N=28)		2-tailed t-test
	Mean	Standard deviation	Mean	Standard deviation	
Left grip strength (kg)	11.2	5.7	6.7	2.1	5.48*
Right grip strength (kg)	11.5	4.6	6.6	5.4	4.97*
Left box and block test (# of blocks)	40.7	17.3	40.0	10.0	0.19
Right box and block test (# of blocks)	40.0	14.2	38.9	11.2	0.33
Left nine hole peg test (sec)	22.7	7.4	20.9	4.5	1.07
Right nine hole peg test (sec)	21.8	8.5	19.6	3.4	1.28

CV t_D 18,26(.95) = 3.28

for the right hand box and block/left hand nine hole peg to − .4727. for the right hand box and block/right hand nine hole peg test.

An inverse correlation was noted between the nine hole peg test results and other variables. The nine hole peg test is measured in seconds, with a higher score indicating poorer performance. Grip strength is measured in kilograms, and the box and block test is measured in the number of blocks moved in a given time period. For both of these tests, the higher the score, the better the performance. Thus, a high negative correlation between the nine hole peg test and the box and block test would indicate that the group would have done well on both tests, or poorly on both tests.

Table 2: Grip Strength and Dexterity Scores of Subjects
with Developmental Disabilities Compared with Norms

2A. Males

Test	Subjects with developmental disabilities			Norm			2-tailed t-test
Left grip strength (kg)	11.2	5.7	28	42.3	12.5	310	+13.03[*]
Right grip strength (kg)	11.5	4.6	28	47.4	12.9	310	14.52[*]
Left box and block test (# of blocks)	40.7	17.3	28	75.4	11.4	310	14.68[*]
Right box and block test (# of blocks)	40.0	14.2	28	76.9	11.6	310	15.80[*]
Left nine hole peg test (sec)	22.7	7.4	28	20.6	3.9	310	-2.48
Right nine hole peg test (sec)	21.8	8.5	28	19.0	3.2	310	-3.64[*]

CV T_d 18,26(.95) = 3.28

2B. Females

Test	Subjects with developmental disabilities			Norm			2-tailed t-test
Left grip strength (kg)	6.7	2.09	28	24.5	7.1	318	13.20[*]
Right grip strength (kg)	6.6	5.4	28	28.5	7.7	318	14.96[*]
Left box and block test (# of blocks)	40.0	10.0	28	75.8	9.5	318	19.03[*]

TABLE 2 (continued)

2B. Females

Test	Subjects with developmental disabilities			Norm			2-tailed t-test
Right box and block test (# of blocks)	38.9	11.1	28	78.4	10.4	318	19.16[*]
Left nine hole peg test (sec)	20.9	4.5	28	19.6	3.4	318	-1.46
Right nine hole peg test (sec)	19.6	3.4	28	17.9	2.8	318	-3.03

CV t_D 18,26 (.95) = 3.28

DISCUSSION

There are a number of limitations to the interpretation of the results. First, the samples were not divided into age groups, but rather were evaluated as a group and compared with norms for the general population. A larger sample would have been conducive to splitting the groups, thus allowing the researchers to do more detailed analyses with specific age groups.

Second, approximately 10% of the subjects were distracted by the colors of the blocks in the box and block test. When they were directed back to the task, they were able to perform, but this probably affected the length of time required for subjects to complete the test. This implies that the dexterity scores may represent differences in cognition rather than truly measuring dexterity which may be a limitation whenever individuals with developmentally delays are tested for manual dexterity.

Dexterity test results indicated no differences between sexes. This does not corroborate the results with normal subjects which have shown that females have slightly better dexterity scores than do males (Mathiowetz et al., 1985b, 1985c). Perhaps childhood physical or sports activities which might account for this difference

Table 3: Correlation between Strength and Dexterity in Subjects with Developmental Disabilities

A. Males

	Right grip strength	Left box and block	Right box and block	Left nine hole peg	Right nine hole peg
Left grip strength	.7445	.7004	.5932	-.5267	-.3678
Right grip strength		.5644	.3794	-.4336	-.2531
Left box and block			.9159	-.7880	-.6240
Right box and block				-.7566	-.5961
Left nine hole peg					.8198

B. Females

	Right grip strength	Left box and block	Right box and block	Left nine hole peg	Right nine hole peg
Left grip strength	.8494	.3668	.3043	-.3941	-.3932
Right grip strength		.4240	.3976	-.3011	-.2594
Left box and block			.8927	-.4727	-.5835
Right box and block				-.5181	-.6405
Left nine hole peg					.5823

in the normal population were not presented or emphasized during growth for this group.

In this study, the grip strength of the males was significantly greater than that of females. This is consistent with the literature based on the normal population (Mathiowetz et al., 1985a) and this may be due to differences in muscle mass between males and females. Lamb (1984) has indicated that size of an individual probably is a factor in strength and ease of movement. The difference may also be due to physiological differences, such as higher androgen levels in males, which may affect the results. (Brooks and Fahey, 1985). It was probably not the result of work experiences since males and females were involved in similar activities during the day.

The grip strength results indicated that normal individuals are stronger than those who are developmentally delayed (Table 2). This supports previous work by other researchers (Morris, Vaughan, and Vaccaro, 1982). Morris et al. (1982), suggested that early planned intervention may improve strength parameters.

Test results for the box and block test demonstrated that our subjects had less dexterity than normal subjects. This may be due to cognitive problems which affect the subject's ability to follow instructions. Down's syndrome children show a significantly lower level of integration of manipulative movements than their non-handicapped peers (Moss and Hogg, 1987). It may also be the result of little practice with these skills. A third possibility is that there is a response delay to changing environmental conditions similar to that noted by Shumway-Cook and Woollacott (1985) during platform perturbations of postural control. If the subjects had difficulty adapting to the tasks, their response times would be slower.

There was no correlation between strength and dexterity variables in females, but there was in males. Further research is needed to examine the relationship between strength and dexterity in this population. It is important to note that therapeutic intervention to improve grip strength will not necessarily affect dexterity abilities. Henry (1968) proposed the specificity hypothesis, which states that motor abilities are specific to a particular task. A high level of strength does not mean a high level of performance on dexterity tasks (Keogh and Sugden, 1985). It is suggested that occupational therapy planned to improve dexterity might focus on dexterity tasks rather than strengthening activities.

The individuals who were subjects in this study may not have been eligible for occupational therapy in their youth. With the adoption of Public Law 94-142, Education of the Handicapped, in 1975, all children were to be educated and related services such as occupational therapy had to be available. Perhaps different results would have been obtained if the population tested had received therapy during their early developmental years. Janicki and Jacobson (1986) found that the older developmentally delayed population (80 years and older) had lower occupational performance skills than the younger group. Their findings suggested that younger individuals may benefit from the provision of active treatment which may not have been available to the elderly group. However, this difference may have been expected based on aging factors. It might be of interest to occupational therapists working with the younger developmentally delayed clients to compare the client's standardized dexterity and grip strength results to those reported in this article.

The poor performance of this group may have implications for the developmentally delayed population in terms of their performance of occupational tasks which require manual dexterity. However, this is conjecture, since no set levels of dexterity have been established for specific tasks, and no validity studies have been done to correlate nine hole peg test and box and block test results with occupational performance tasks. Mathiowetz et al. (1985b, 1985c) recommended care in interpreting box and block and nine hole peg test results since they are broad screening tests.

The measurement of treatment outcomes in occupational therapy among the developmentally disabled population is limited by the lack of standardized assessments available for use with this population. Dexterity testing and grip strength measurements are often used in the clinic, but interpretation of assessments is inconclusive because of the lack of normative performance information for this group.

In evaluating strength and dexterity of adults with retardation, results are compared to norms established on adults without pathology. However, this comparison ignores the differences that are present among individuals with developmental disabilities. Therapists do not have specific guidelines to determine how the individuals in this group may compare to their peers who are developmentally delayed. That is, there may be difficulty with dexterity as a result of the problem of the developmental delay, rather than a problem specifically with dexterity.

There may be two overlapping normal distributions of scores, one for individuals with developmental disabilities and a second one for the general population. Future study, by testing a larger sample of the population with developmental delays might help determine if there is a difference for the group as a whole when compared to the population as a whole. This might then provide therapists with reasonable expectations for their clients, based on data which were gathered for the general population with developmental disabilities.

The present study was done to analyze grip strength and dexterity in a group of individuals with developmental disabilities. There were differences noted between the subjects and the general population. Therapists who treat individuals with developmental delays might evaluate their clients with these data in mind and compare their clients to these values. Although there were not enough subjects in this study to consider these data as norms for the developmentally delayed population, they may be guidelines for the expectations of therapists who work with clients with developmental delays. It may also be important in recommending individuals for sheltered workshop placement to note that the strength and dexterity of the clients may not be within normal limits.

The second major finding is that there were not high correlations between grip strength and measures of dexterity in this group. Therapists who treat clients for dexterity and strength problems need to remember that working with one aspect of hand function, such as grip strength will not necessarily lead to improvement in another area, such as fine hand dexterity. It is recommended that therapists need to consider not only testing, but also treating the problems of both grip strength and dexterity.

REFERENCES

Brook, G. A. & Fahey, T. D. (1985). *Exercise physiology: Human bioenergetics and its application*. New York: MacMillan Publishing Co.

Henry, F. M. (1968). Specificity versus generality in learning motor skill. In R.C. Brown and G.S. Kenyon (Eds.) *Classical studies on physical activity*. Englewood Cliffs, N.J.: Prentice-Hall.

Janicki, M. P. & Jacobson, J. W. (1986). General trends in sensory, physical, and behavioral abilities among older mentally retarded persons. *American Journal of Mental Deficiency*, *90*, 490-500.

Keogh, J. & Sugden, D. (1985). *Movement skill development*. New York: MacMillan Publishing Co.

Lamb, D. R. (1984). *Physiology of exercise*. New York: MacMillan Publishing Co.

Mathiowetz, V., Kashman, N., Volland, G., Weber, K., Dowe, M., & Rogers, S. (1985a). Grip and pinch strength: normative data for adults. *Archives of Physical Medicine and Rehabilitation*, *66*, 69-72.

Mathiowetz, V., Volland, G., Kashman, N., & Weber, K., (1985b). Adult norms for the box and block test of manual dexterity. *American Journal of Occupational Therapy*, *39*(6), 386-391.

Mathiowetz, V., Weber, K., Kashman, N., & Volland, G., (1985c). Adult norms for the nine hole peg test of finger dexterity. *Occupational Therapy Journal of Research*, *5*(1), 25-38.

Morris, A. F., Vaghan, S. E., & Vaccaro (1982). Measurements of neuromuscular tone and strength in Down's syndrome children. *Journal of Mental Deficiency Research*, *26*, 41-46.

Moss, S., & Hogg, J. (1987). The integration of manipulative movements in children with Down's syndrome and their non-handicapped peers. *Human Movement Science*, *6*, 67-99.

Shumway-Cook, A., & Woollacott, M. H. (1985). Dynamics of postural control in the child with Down syndrome. *Physical Therapy*, *65*(9), 1315-1322.

Occupational Therapy in Operation Outreach: Community Based Approach to Adapted Positioning Equipment

Janet D. Stout, MS, OTR
Judy Atkins, OTR
Carolyn Hamann, OTR

SUMMARY. A mobile outreach program is presented here as a response to the rapidly expanding demand for occupational therapy services in the field of developmental disabilities. Historical overview of Operation Outreach will include discussion of societal trends influencing the program as well as factual information specific to the Indiana University (IU) experience. Demand for increased productivity and efficiency with cost containment led to IU's modified truck, housing a complete mobile adapted equipment laboratory, for convenient on-site evaluations and service of wheelchairs and custom designed positioning equipment. Operation Outreach was designed for the developmentally disabled to help address the needs of the whole person in his own environment, to enhance wellness, and to improve quality of life.

Janet Stout is an assistant professor in the occupational therapy program at Indiana University School of Medicine, Indianapolis, IN 46223. Judy Atkins and Carolyn Hamann are supervisor and assistant supervisor, respectively, in the Occupational Therapy Department at the James Whitcomb Riley Hospital for Children, Indiana University Hospitals, Indianapolis, IN 46223.

The authors would like to express thanks to Celestine Hamant and Pat Griswold for their valuable assistance and support, and to Anita Slominski for the vision and wisdom to focus on the patients' needs in a changing world of medicine. Sincere appreciation is also extended to the Riley Cheer Guild Association, and to the Indiana University Hospitals. Without their support this outreach program would not have been possible.

HISTORICAL OVERVIEW

The United States Department of Health, Education and Welfare (now called the Department of Health and Human Services) recognized almost 20 years ago a trend toward decentralization in delivery of rehabilitation services. Its 1969 report indicated that rehabilitation enterprise in the United States at that time was essentially a centralized service delivery system. "Although occasional attempts are made to bring the service closer to the consumer, remoteness and disassociation from clients still are more common than localization and community contiguity."

The report also expounded on the problem associated with geographical maldistribution of services, pointing out that "the more centralized the system, the greater will be the number of disabled persons who have to inconvenience themselves substantially to establish communication with the helping source." The one children's hospital in Indiana was an example, being centrally located in Indianapolis and requiring up to a four hour drive for clients in outlying areas to reach the hospital.

As a result of the national decentralization trend, legislation in the state of Indiana resulted in development of community based care centers for the developmentally disabled. The resulting pediatric nursing home concept allowed children and adults to be returned to their communities and closer to their families' homes. Often being incorporated into local school, work, recreational, and camp programs, these developmentally disabled children and adults require adapted seating to enhance their community independence. State schools had provided some clients with adapted seating which needed continued monitoring.

Turning from the past to look at perspectives on the future, Taira (1985) states

> The escalating costs of hospital care have been the primary incentives for moving patients out of acute settings and thus increasing the need for occupational therapy services in the community. Yet, relatively few therapists have moved from the medical model even though the need exists and the legislation encourages that service be provided in the least restrictive alternative.

Shannon (1985) supports community based practice stating,

> Given the holistic perspective of the profession, its broad
> knowledge base and technology built upon the requirements
> for daily living, occupational therapy has a unique opportunity
> to strengthen its viability in the community and ultimately, its
> viability in promoting a more healthy society.

THE INDIANA UNIVERSITY EXPERIENCE

Responsiveness to consumer needs in the 1970s required a creative approach from the occupational therapists treating the community based population. Operation Outreach at Indiana University
was initiated in the 1970s by the movement of hospital based programs with a view toward the community. Indiana University therapists began consulting in pediatric nursing homes in 1974 and provided inservices for nurses, teachers, and therapists who previously
had been working primarily with the geriatric population. After
much preparatory planning, a pilot project was launched in 1978
when registered occupational therapists (OTRs), from the James
Whitcomb Riley Hospital for Children and the Cerebral Palsy
Clinic at Indiana University Medical Center, began going to two
pediatric nursing home facilities (one skilled care facility with 150
beds and one intermediate care facility with 75 beds). This marked
a significant change from previous practice requiring patient attendance at the hospital for all wheelchair and positioning needs.

Initially a team consisting of a registered occupational therapist
(OTR), and an adapted equipment technician traveled in a university owned vehicle carrying equipment and supplies in cardboard
boxes. They were only able to handle evaluations, minor repairs
and deliveries due to limitations in equipment, supplies, and space,
but several advantages were evident compared to hospital based
treatment. Direct communication was possible between therapist
and primary caregivers. Patients were not exhausted by travel and
therefore provided a truer picture for positioning evaluations. Issues
other than equipment, such as behavior problems or feeding and
grooming difficulties, could be addressed by seeing the children in
their own environment.

As the demand for the outreach services grew to include more patients and other facilities, the borrowed vehicle and limited equipment became less conducive to efficiency. However, by this time those involved had a vision of expanding the program goals to include evaluating, managing, and providing more complete services to individuals in the intrastate area. The apparent need for expanded services was researched and documented.

Societal trends of disease prevention and wellness, community based care, and desire for cost containment in health care strengthened the case for Operation Outreach's expansion to include a special mobile unit. Wellness included all people, regardless of the presence of chronic disabling conditions (White, 1981) and therefore was relevant to the nursing home population. Disease prevention was addressed by Operation Outreach because early diagnosis and remediation could be accomplished through the program to prevent more serious or permanently disabling conditions resulting from poor positioning.

Environmental factors, as Johnson (1986) pointed out, are important in considering an individual's total condition, giving credibility to seeing clients in their own settings. Escalating health care costs led to increasing demands upon health care systems to provide productive and efficient services while containing costs, which Operation Outreach does. The program recognizes Johnson's (1977) challenge "to set forth our goals clearly and coherently, and to act on our convictions recognizing that it is not only possible but necessary to join humanitarianism and accountability."

MOBILE POSITIONING LABORATORY

The Indiana University Hospitals' Mobile Positioning Laboratory Unit began service in May, 1988, turning Outreach vision into reality (Photo 1). The unit consists of a 6 passenger pick-up truck with attached 5th wheel trailer equipped with drill press, band saw, sander, grinder, table saw, wheelchair tie downs, hand tools, work bench, and storage compartments for stock (Photo 2). The unit is both heated for winter and air conditioned for summer. Community facilities involved in the program have installed a special electrical outlet on the outside of their facilities, where the mobile unit has access to necessary electrical supply.

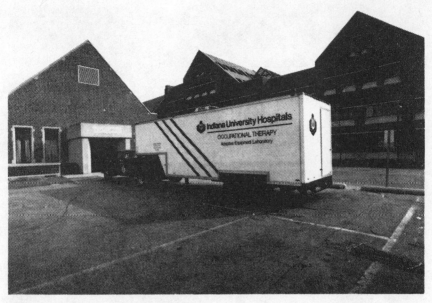

PHOTO 1

Settings and populations served by the mobile lab are varied. The seventeen settings currently involved include five educational (school) programs, three adult nursing homes, and nine pediatric nursing homes and serve a total of 690 persons having a wide variety of diagnoses. The sites, located all over Indiana, are visited 2-10 times per year.

To ensure continuity of care each site has a designated team of 1-2 OTRs, 1 Certified Occupational Therapy Assistant (COTA), and 2-3 adapted equipment technicians. A total of 10 OTRs, 2 COTAs, 6 equipment technicians from Indiana University Hospitals as well as OT affiliate students spend part of their time involved with Operation Outreach. Staff involved in the program have received special driver's training to manage the unit, which is similar to a small semitractor-trailer. Employees are covered by workman's compensation and insurance on the visits just as they are when working in the hospital. Facility personnel are responsible for providing a list of patient concerns and equipment problems to occupational ther-

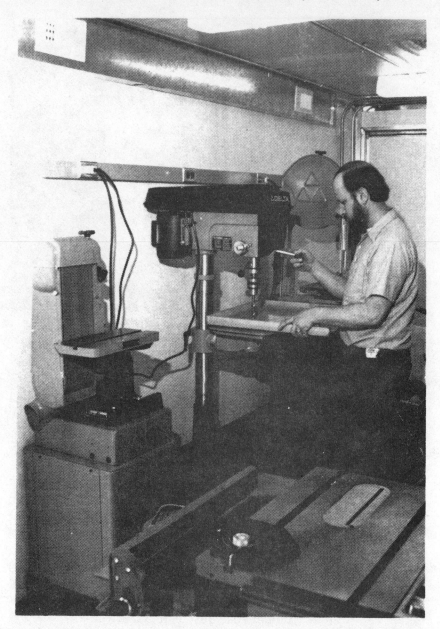

PHOTO 2

apy 4-6 weeks prior to outreach dates to increase efficient provision of needed repairs or replacements on the day of the visit.

Bringing this service on site benefits the facility and its residents in the following ways:

- — allows for identification of clients needing services, not previously referred;
- — improves communication with primary caretakers;
- — eliminates travel stress for the residents;
- — decreases delays in provision of service; ·
- — decreases transportation costs of residents coming for equipment checks;
- — decreases paperwork for the facility;
- — provides complete positioning evaluation/service on site, including linear designs as well as foam-in-place seating systems; and
- — maximizes convenience.

A secondary benefit is that there is more room for patients being treated in the overcrowded hospital department due to the decreased number of patients transported from other facilities. Patients still come to the hospital for medical care since positioning is only one part of their comprehensive healthcare.

Measuring results monetarily, it is estimated that each trip saves taxpayers $2,000-$10,000 depending upon the distance traveled and the number of patients or students seen. Travel costs are divided among the 15-20 residents or students seen per visit, but they are far less than the average cost of transporting each client (usually by ambulance) to the medical center and paying for the aide to accompany them. Patients are charged as out-patients, just as any home visit would be. Many of the patients are on Medicaid and/or Medicare. Some are on Crippled Children's Funding, and still others may have private insurance. All of these funding sources have been supportive of this program. Funding of the equipped mobile unit was provided through Indiana University Hospitals and the Riley Cheer Guild. Both are examples of community generosity for a worthwhile project.

CASE STUDIES

Each handicapped individual and his equipment are carefully evaluated by skilled IU Hospital occupational therapists and adapted equipment technicians. By seeing the person in his own environment and by talking with the people who actually provide his care each day, Operation Outreach staff members learn about the individual and his disability. They observe first-hand the kinds of activities he performs and the special problems he encounters in his everyday routine. Chairs are always adjusted or modified to fit the child or adult's own measurements so they provide safety, mobility and maximum comfort.

Case Study #1

James R. is an 18-year old with a diagnosis of spina bifida (unrepaired) and hydrocephalus. He was initially seen at age 9 years on an Outreach visit to his facility. Because of his unrepaired bifida, he had spent the first 9 years of his life in a prone position.

During an on site visit the facility staff brought this client to the attention of the evaluation team, feeling that cognitively he could handle more of his own care if he could be positioned more optimally. Following evaluation and consultation with orthopedics and neurosurgery, James was positioned upright. After being positioned with proper support and pressure relief, he could then propel himself, feed himself, and attend school.

Through increased communication with the facility staff, they brought this child to the attention of the Outreach staff. Prior to the visits to the facility, they were unaware that this service was available to clients like James R. This child was given a new life perspective as a direct result of Operation Outreach.

Case Study #2

Shannon S. is a 7-year-old female with a diagnosis of cerebral palsy spastic quadriplegia. She had been followed in the occupational therapy department, requiring numerous trips and time away from work for her mother. When the question of placement for Shannon arose, it was comforting to the mother that Shannon could have her equipment needs met at the nursing home. Shannon's mother was invited to visit on outreach days and to continue to have communication with the therapists. In this case the therapist who had followed the patient prior to placement is the same one serving the residential facility, preserving continuity of care and enhancing rapport with the family and the facility.

CONCLUSION

Medical, legislative, and societal trends toward community based practice and cost containment led to the current Indiana University Occupational Therapy Outreach Program. The program expanded from visiting 2 sites using a borrowed vehicle and boxed hand tools to the current fully equipped truck and trailer. The 17 facilities currently involved and third party payers have been supportive of the project and its benefits of quality care and cost containment.

REFERENCES

Johnson, J.A. (1968). Wellness and Occupational Therapy. *The American Journal of Occupational Therapy, 40*, 753-758.

Johnson, J.A. (1977). Humanitarianism and accountability: A challenge for occupational therapy on its 60th anniversary. *The American Journal of Occupational Therapy, 31*, 631-637.

Rusalem, H. & Baxt, R. (1969). *Delivering rehabilitation services*. Washington, DC: U.S. Department of Health Education and Welfare.

Shannon, P.D. (1985). From another perspective: An overview of the issue. *Occupational Therapy in Health Care, 2*, No. 1, p. 11.

Tiara, E.D. (1985). After treatment what? Roles for occupational therapists in community. *Occupational Therapy in Health Care, 2*, No. 1, p. 13.

White, V.K. (1986). Promoting health and wellness: A theme for the eighties. *The American Journal of Occupational Therapy, 40*, 743-748.

The Importance of Program Evaluation: Introduction to the Evaluation of a Community Program for Developmentally Disabled Adults

Julie Shaperman, MS, MA, OTR, FAOTA

Objective documentation of patient progress in occupational therapy is required by payment agencies and administrators; this has become an increasingly important part of our work. We often hear our colleagues express the wish that they had the time and knew how to do some studies to show that their program is really producing positive results in the day-to-day treatment of patients. Yet, few clinicians can organize and conduct the kind of group comparison studies that would be needed.

One practical way to document program effects is to incorporate an evaluation into the design of the occupational therapy program. This could demonstrate that the program was, in fact, achieving stated objectives and, at the same time, it could convince administrators that our services are of measurable benefit to patients.

There is some risk in conducting a program evaluation, however. It might *not* demonstrate that the program is as effective as we believe it is. Yet, negative findings may be as valuable to the program's development as positive findings if we use the information creatively to improve the program. We should not fear a negative result; the therapists have not failed; the program just needs revision.

Recently, a very innovative community program for developmentally disabled adults was evaluated by an outside agency as a condition of its grant funding. The accompanying article describes the evaluation of this community program. The evaluation showed that the program did not meet its stated objectives. The staff members were convinced that they were providing good service to their patients. Although they were disappointed in the results of the evaluation, it gave them an opportunity to revise and improve the program. Then, the evaluation's findings served as a basis for comparison when the revised program was evaluated. The staff realized that the stated objectives were beyond anything that could be expected under the circumstances in which the program operated. The result was a more realistic set of objectives that were achievable and measurable.

The program evaluation revealed some other findings that helped streamline program procedures. For example, the evaluation identified some characteristics of persons in both populations (elderly and developmentally disabled) which were associated with successful home helper partnerships. The evaluation demonstrated the relative effectiveness of various methods of orienting the older persons in ways of supervising their developmentally disabled helpers. The evaluation also revealed an important conceptual flaw in the program: most elderly people who are at risk for placement in a nursing home are too ill to be able to supervise a developmentally disabled helper. The helper might give some respite to the primary caregiver, but the help would not be sufficient to delay institutionalization, if that was imminent.

There are many ways of conducting program evaluations; they extend from a very informal self-assessment to a highly formalized study by an outside organization. The methodology of the evaluation described here followed several steps:

1. state each program objective;
2. list the activities of the program to meet each objective;
3. decide on a standard or level of achievement for each activity/ goal;
4. restate each standard as a research question;
5. define a methodology for answering each research question considering design, sample, measuring instruments along with their reliability and validity as well as threats to validity of the study; and
6. whenever possible, blend the measures and schedules of the

evaluation into those of the program so the program will not be changed by the evaluation procedures.

There are many programs offered to developmentally disabled adults today to enhance their employability and decrease the cost of their public support. Many such programs end in disappointment for the participants as well as for the program developers. We need to understand what kinds of services will really help developmentally disabled people achieve their greatest potential. The description of the evaluation is offered as a stimulus to clinicians to incorporate objective evaluation mechanisms into programs you conduct. The findings, negative or positive, will strengthen the program. It is hoped that some of the methods used in this program evaluation will be useful in other community based programs.

An Exchange of Services Program for Adults with Developmental Disabilities: How Effective Was It?

Julie Shaperman, MS, MA, OTR, FAOTA
Charles E. Lewis, MD, ScD

SUMMARY. A randomized controlled trial was conducted to evaluate a community program to train, match and place developmentally disabled adults with elderly people who needed help with housekeeping, personal care and companionship. Program goals were not achieved, as employment of persons with developmental disabilities did not increase and institutionalization of elderly people was not delayed. The program did improve feelings of well-being. Program costs exceeded $200 per person-month. Attrition was high, and survival analysis identified critical periods for retention in the program.

INTRODUCTION

There is considerable concern over the consequences of inappropriate institutionalization of individuals. It is not surprising, there-

---

Julie Shaperman is a research occupational therapist at UCLA, formerly in the Department of General Internal Medicine, currently in the Department of Pediatrics. Charles E. Lewis is Chief, Department of General Internal Medicine, and Professor of Medicine, Public Health and Nursing, University of California, Los Angeles.

The authors are grateful to Frederick J. Dorey, PhD, Senior Statistician, UCLA School of Medicine, for valuable assistance in statistical analysis of data.

Address correspondence to: Julie Shaperman, UCLA Rehabilitation Center 25-26, 1000 Veteran Avenue, Los Angeles, CA 90024-1653.

The opinions, conclusions, and proposals in the text are those of the author and do not necessarily represent the views of the Robert Wood Johnson Foundation.

241

fore, that a proposal for providing work-training for mentally retarded adults prior to placement with aged individuals in need of housekeeping and other support services evoked considerable interest. The ultimate goal of the program was to prevent premature institutionalization of persons in both groups and to promote paid employment of mentally retarded persons. It was suggested that the matching of two partially disabled persons to augment each contributor could have a potentially synergising effect in which each might gain more than he or she contributed to the partnership.

Such an effort, the Companion Program, received initial support in 1981 from the California Department of Rehabilitation. An effort to expand the program and develop a model for generalized use was funded by the Robert Wood Johnson Foundation between 1983 and 1986, with the condition that it be evaluated by an independent outside agency. The authors conducted the evaluation in the form of a randomized controlled trial with measures before and after participation in the program of certain dimensions in both groups of participants. The evaluators did not plan or operate the program, so this paper focuses primarily on the evaluation.

The program had strong intuitive appeal, so it was surprising when it did not demonstrate its effectiveness. Negative results can provide very useful information for future program development if we understand the reasons a program has failed, however. The program under evaluation was not an occupational therapy program, but the evaluation methods, findings and analysis are very relevant to occupational therapy.

The evaluation determined whether the program met its objectives. The general objective was to match elderly people with persons with mental retardation and other developmental disabilities so they would help each other live independently in the community. Specific program objectives were: (1) to train developmentally disabled adults in skills that would increase employability; (2) to decrease institutional care experiences of elderly persons by providing personal care, housekeeping and/or companionship at no cost; (3) to improve the sense of well-being in both groups; (4) to decrease consumption of community and public services among persons in both groups and thus demonstrate cost effectiveness of the program.

EVALUATION DESIGN AND METHODOLOGY

The evaluation was a randomized controlled trial with lagged control group. Experimental subjects started participating in the program immediately; control subjects waited six months. The waiting time served as a control period, after which the program was offered to those in the control group. A new cohort started every ten weeks and the study extended over a two and one-half year period. Program staff members recruited all persons for the program; evaluation staff randomly assigned them to experimental or control status. Evaluation measures were administered to all persons in both groups at entry and after six months.

Subjects

The study included 93 developmentally disabled adults, called companions, and 99 elderly people, called seniors. Companions' ages ranged from 18 to 61 years with a mean of 28 for both experimental and control groups. There were 53 females and 40 males. Counselors and teachers referred three-fourths of the companions to the program. Over half lived with their families; another third lived alone or with a roommate and a small number lived in group homes.

At the time the companions entered the program, they said their primary reason for participating was to help other people (48% of applicants), to learn new skills (18 percent), to get job-related experience (14 percent), to get companionship (12 percent) and for other reasons (8 percent). At enrollment, 75 percent of companions had no major medical condition; the other 25 percent had conditions such as blindness, deafness, arthritis or cerebral palsy. Three-fourths of the applicants reported that they received income supplements such as supplemental security income (SSI) or social security disability payments, and they received health care coverage through MediCal or Medicare.

Program staff members established the following criteria for admission to the program: desire to participate in all aspects of the program; ability to follow instructions and perform tasks under supervision; permission from family; ability to travel to training and work site; ability to lift 25 pounds; absence of antisocial behavior, substance abuse and seizures. The sample comprised a mild to moderately developmentally disabled group of people who lived in the southwestern area of Los Angeles County.

The average ages of seniors in the program were 75 years for the experimental group and 74 years for the control group; the age range was from 55 to 96 years. There were 75 females and 24 males. Sixty percent of seniors heard of the program from counselors, professional caregivers and through affiliation with community groups. Twenty-five percent lived alone; 38 percent lived with a spouse and others lived with other family members or caregivers. The seniors enrolled in the program primarily to get help with housekeeping (44 percent of applicants), personal care (31 percent), and companionship (25 percent).

Almost all seniors reported some major medical condition; these included heart disease, arthritis, diabetes, cancer and/or stroke. Fewer than 20 percent of seniors received any type of publicly funded income supplement, but 85 percent of experimental and 93 percent of control subjects had health care coverage through Medicare and/or MediCal. Seniors reported using a large variety of other assistance provided mostly by family members, friends or persons hired to work in the house or yard. Except for health services, the seniors were *not* large consumers of community and public services.

Program staff members accepted seniors into the program if they wished to participate, lived in the area, could supervise (or had someone else who could supervise) the companion, could provide a meal in exchange for each work period, and did not have a history of substance abuse or antisocial behavior. Staff members told seniors that the companions were developmentally disabled and that meant they were slow learners.

The Program

Companions received training three half-days a week for six to ten weeks. Training included housekeeping skills, personal care procedures, information on aging and basic safety practices. Seniors joined the companions for two to six orientation sessions. One-third of the seniors could not attend group sessions and they were oriented at home. The program staff then matched seniors and companions, arranged exchange-of-service agreements and monitored partnerships. Matching was based on needs of seniors, skills of companions, personality factors, personal preferences and practical considerations such as timing, location and availability. Companions worked a few hours a week in exchange for a meal, but they received no money.

The Evaluation

Data were gathered from interviews and administration of relevant instruments at enrollment and after six months. Companions' parents or counselors and the program staff also provided data on companions. Evaluators monitored the type and duration of each person's participation in the program as a measure of the amount of service received; these data were recorded on life tables to measure the "survival" of each person and partnership. Finally, the evaluators interviewed each person at the time he or she left the program.

Evaluation instruments were selected for reliability, validity and the availability of normative data. For companions, the Behavior Development Survey (Pawlarczk & Schumacher, 1983; Research Group, 1979) provided community norms for adults with various levels of mental retardation. The survey is a shortened version of the Adaptive Behavior Scale developed by the American Association on Mental Deficiency. The survey has subscales on Community Self-Sufficiency, Personal-Social Responsibility, Social Adaptation and Social Living which were of particular interest. As a reliability measure, twelve items from the survey were formulated into a standardized performance measure; item scores correlated with survey responses in a range from .69 to .86.

For seniors, the Sickness Impact Profile (Bergner et al., 1976) was used to measure functional status. The Lawton Morale Scale (Lawton et al., 1982) and the Rand General Well-Being (Veit & Ware, 1983) and Rand Social Activities Scales (Donald & Ware, 1982) developed and standardized in the national Health Insurance Experiment were used. Health status was recorded on a questionnaire which was a slightly shortened form of one used in the UCLA Medical Ambulatory Care Clinic. Resource utilization measures were developed for the evaluation; inter-rater reliability for that instrument reached a correlation of .78.

Items on the companions' resource utilization questionnaire identified previous school, work training and employment experiences, services from counselors at regional centers, vocational rehabilitation agency services, health insurance coverage, income supplements, frequency of physician visits, help with shopping or transportation, housing arrangements and informal supports such as social clubs and help from family and friends. The seniors' resource utilization questionnaire identified similar data but included more detail on health services and community aid. Each resource area included questions on who provided the help, the amount of help each person currently used and how it was paid for.

Finally, semi-structured interviews provided information on expectations at enrollment and satisfaction after six months. Control subjects described their activities and substitute services during the control period. Exit interviews were conducted by telephone; these concerned experiences while in the program, alternate services people planned to use and suggestions for ways to improve the program. Since evaluators were not program staff members; people leaving the program were very candid in discussing their experiences.

Data Analysis

Three types of data were examined. First the life table data on types and amounts of participation proved very important because there was high attrition. Statistical survival analysis (computer program BMD P1L) was used to determine critical periods for leaving the program in relation to program events such as enrollment, training, orientation and placement. The life table data provided a total number of person-months of service that clients received. Total program costs divided by the number of person-months of service defined the cost per person-month of program operation. A second data set provided a comparison of program effects on experimentals versus controls. These data were first examined using descriptive statistics, and t tests or chi square analyses were used to indicate levels of significance. A stepwise regression analysis was also done to define the characteristics of persons in relation to the time they left the program (computer program BMD P2L). Finally, a content analysis of the qualitative data on expectations, satisfaction and leaving the program was done.

RESULTS

Survival Analysis and Program Effects

The survival analysis demonstrated a statistically significant difference in overall survival distributions for companions versus seniors (P = .005). Companions had a median survival probability of 23 weeks at enrollment (median survival provides a measure of the half life of the group or is when half of the group at risk has left the program). Median survival, or retention, increased to 29 weeks if companions entered training and to 43 weeks if they completed training. After that, retention increased gradually as the number of persons at risk of leaving declined. The critical period for companions to leave the program was the end of training; if they entered a partnership, retention increased markedly.

In contrast, the start and end of senior orientation were critical times for them to leave the program. There was a sharp drop in seniors' survival distributions just after starting the program. Seniors' median survival probability at enrollment was only six weeks. Table 1 shows survival probabilities for companions and seniors at critical program times; Figure 1 shows survival distributions for both populations.

The large attrition affected the evaluation of program effects on experimental versus control subjects. Only 57 percent of companions and 45 percent of seniors stayed long enough to be in a partnership. By the time of the six-month evaluation the number of companion experimental subjects decreased from 51 to 30 (a loss of 41 percent) and the number of seniors decreased from 56 to 22 (a loss of 60 percent).

Comparisons on the principal measures employed in the evalua-

Table 1.

Conditional Survival Probabilities for Companions and Seniors

If Companion Survives Until:	Probability of Surviving Until:					Median Survival
	3 weeks	6 weeks	3 months	6 months	1 year	
Program enrollment	.85	.73	.60	.45	.27	23 weeks
Training starts	-	.87	.70	.53	.28	29 weeks
Training ends	-	-	-	.60	.46	43 weeks
In partnership 10 wks.	-	-	-	.85	.49	47 weeks
If Senior Survives Until:						
Program enrollment	.59	.47	.39	.29	.19	6 weeks
Orientation starts	-	.78	.61	.46	.35	22 weeks
Orientation ends	-	-	.78	.59	.44	46 weeks
In partnership 10 wks.	-	-	.87	.66	.49	49 weeks

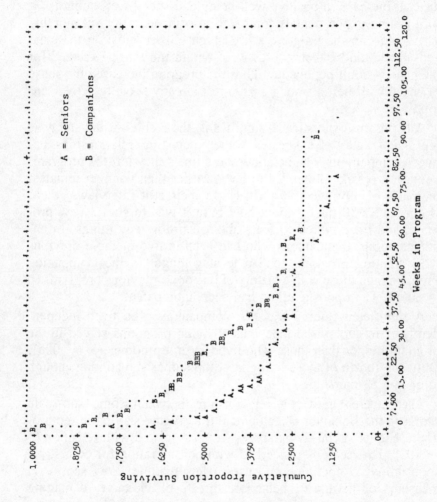

Figure 1. Cumulative Survival Distribution of Seniors and Companions

249

tion among the remaining 30 companions and 22 senior experimentals and their controls indicated that there was little difference that could be attributed to program participation. Seniors showed a significant increase in positive well-being and social well-being ($p <$ .05) among experimentals compared to controls, after six months. The seniors in the program scored high on participation in social activities initially; their scores were within the range expected for the general adult population. Thus the program increased the sense of social well-being among a group of already socially active seniors.

Although not statistically significant, the results of the stepwise regression analysis suggested some interesting relationships between companions' characteristics and times they left the program. Females over age 30 tended to leave earlier than younger females, or males of any age ($p = .054$). In their exit interviews, these women over 30 talked about how hard it was to start a new program, and they expressed fears about learning new things. In another finding, companions who had been in two or more previous work training programs tended to stay longer in the Companion Program than those with a history of one or no previous programs ($p = .058$). The opposite effect had been anticipated.

A significant finding was that companions who lived independently or in supervised independent living programs stayed in the program longer than those who lived in group homes ($p = .025$). Only one-fourth of those living in group homes stayed long enough to be in a partnership.

There were significant relationships between some sub-scale scores in the Behavior Development Survey and staying in the program. Higher social living scores were associated with retention ($p = .02$). This scale is concerned with consideration for others, responsibility, cooperation and use of leisure time. Low scores on measures of disruptive behavior, threats of violence, damaging property, use of profane language, rebelliousness and untrustworthiness were associated with retention ($p = .05$). These two sub-scales were correlated ($r = -.49$) suggesting that higher social living scores and fewer maladaptive behaviors are associated with retention, as would be expected.

Reasons for Termination

Since attrition was such a major issue in the evaluation, the interviews at enrollment concerning expectations, the six-month interviews for those who stayed, and the exit interviews for those who left were examined carefully. At enrollment, the primary reasons companions joined the program was to help another person. On leaving, companions talked primarily about the kind of work they had to do; the idea of helping others paled in comparison to the tasks they had to perform (and which represented giving help). Table 2 lists companions' reasons for leaving the program.

The companions who were terminated by staff members showed inappropriate behavior during training. Companions who disliked the work or their senior usually said they disliked housework; or complained that the seniors made unreasonable demands. If the senior dismissed the companion, it was especially traumatic and the companion was hesitant to risk another placement. The dissatisfied companions spoke only of the tasks involved and rarely mentioned their primary reason for joining the program to help another person. In contrast, companions who stayed six months and were satisfied with the program spoke more about the relationship with the senior than about the tasks they performed.

One program objective was to increase employment among companions. Two companions (4 percent of experimentals) left the program to take paid jobs. One had the job before joining the program and left because the program interfered with the job. The other companion took additional training and was later employed as a personal care attendant. There was no significant difference between numbers of companions in the experimental versus the control group who became employed, and no difference in the number who continued to receive public support payments.

Seniors who left the program soon after enrollment said that they did not think a developmentally disabled person would be able to help them. Those who left after a period in a partnership often cited excessive amounts of supervision that companions required. Those who stayed in the program and were satisfied at six months talked about how hard the companions tried to please them and how much they liked the companions. Although satisfied seniors said compan-

Table 2.

Reasons Companions Left the Program

N = 78

	When Companions Left**					
Reason for Leaving	T 1	T 2	T 3	T 4	T 5	Total
Changed their mind, no transportation or bored with program.	11	4	0	0	0	15 (19)*
Terminated by staff	0	4	5	0	6	15 (19)
Prefer other program	6	6	0	1	3	16 (21)
Got a job	0	1	2	2	3	8 (10)
Dislike the work or dislike their senior	1	1	3	3	13	21 (27)
Illness	0	1	0	1	1	3 (04)
Total No. of Companions	18	17	10	7	26	78 (100)

* Column percentages

** Times companions left the program

T 1 Before training

T 2 During training

T 3 Before placement

T 4 Partner 10 weeks or less

T 5 Over 10 weeks as partner

ions were helpful to them, most seniors needed help for tasks that were beyond the skill level of the companions. There was no evidence that companion services lessened the amount of other services the seniors needed.

Another program objective was to decrease the experience of seniors with institutional care. Five percent of experimental and control subjects did go to nursing homes, so there was not significant difference between groups on that measure. Also, review of characteristics of seniors in the program showed that few seniors in the program were at risk for institutionalization (Branch & Jette, 1982; Kraus et al., 1976). Seniors sick enough to be at risk could not supervise a companion and were not in the program.

Program Costs

First, costs were allocated to senior or companion services in relation to the program's operating pattern. Next, the total expense for each group was divided by the number of person-months shown in the life tables. The cost per companion-month was $218. and the cost per senior-month was $204. The cost per partnership-month was $422. Few companions worked more than ten hours per week, so these costs must be considered in relation to the services provided.

DISCUSSION

Program Objectives

The results indicate that program participation did not achieve the general objectives of increasing employability of companions or delaying institutionalization of seniors. Participation was associated with improved feelings of well-being among seniors; no other program effects were detected. The program was not cost effective; there was no offset effect from lowering costs of other services and the program cost over $200 per person-month for each participant with the only measured benefit being improved well-being among seniors. The large attrition in both groups suggests that there was considerable dissatisfaction with the program. Those in both groups who stayed had higher scores in social living and social activities and their participation increased this socialization. Thus, the program was aptly named the "Companion Program."

In retrospect, closer examination of risk factors for institutionalization would have revealed that prevention of this phenomenon requires the provision of rather complex support services. Similarly, analysis of the work capacities of most developmentally disabled adults would have suggested that even with a reasonable period of training, these services are generally beyond their capacity unless they are closely supervised.

It was also not reasonable to expect developmentally disabled adults and their families to renounce the security of monthly support under SSI without the assurance that they could return to their level of disability support in the event their paid employment attempt failed. Programs that offer supported employment address this problem to some extent.

The program staff saw the enthusiasm of the companions as a commitment to the program, but this enthusiasm faded with time. The companions did not see themselves in the worker role and could not make the transition to that occupational role without interventions and support for that kind of change. Occupational therapy input might have made a difference in the companions' participation in the program.

Evaluation Methods

Randomized controlled trials are not frequently used in the evaluation of occupational therapy programs in the community, but this study demonstrates important benefits of this design. First, findings indicated that most participants improved during their six-month participation in the program. It would be natural to conclude that the program had been highly beneficial to them except that the control subjects improved just as much as those in the experimental groups. Without a randomly assigned control group for comparison, one could be misled into believing that changes over time were related to program participation.

A concern voiced over the use of control groups in such programs is denial of service to the control group. With the lag design, all persons were offered service. It did not appear that the delay in receiving services had an adverse affect on controls; they made other arrangements during the waiting period.

Survival analysis proved to be a very useful method of analyzing attrition; it identified critical periods for seniors and companions to leave the program so staff members could examine program procedures at those times. This method may prove useful in other cost-benefit studies.

CONCLUSION

The partnerships between developmentally disabled adults and elderly people to provide mutual support, delay institutionalization and promote paid employment of developmentally disabled people did not prove beneficial except to promote the feeling of well-being. The partnerships did not produce significantly more than each person brought to the program originally. Agencies concerned with promoting these outcomes need to conduct or support evaluations of the programs they sponsor so that the programs result in long term change, personal growth and improved quality of life for their clients.

REFERENCES

Bergner, M., Bobbitt, R.A., Pollard, W.E., Martin, D.P., & Gilson, B.S. (1976). The Sickness Impact Profile: Validation of a health status measure. Medical Care, 14, 57-67.

Branch, L.G., & Jette, A.M. (1982). A prospective study of long-term-care institutionalization among the aged. American Journal of Public Health, 72, 1373-1379.

Donald, C.A., & Ware, J.E. Jr. (1982). The quantification of social contacts and resources. Santa Monica: RAND Corporation, R-2937-HHS.

Kraus, A., Spasoff, R., & Beattie, E. (1976). Elderly applicants to long-term care institutions. Journal of the American Geriatric Society, 24, 117-125.

Lawton, M.P., Moss, M., Fulcomer, M., & Kleban, M.H. (1982). A research and service-oriented multilevel assessment instrument. Journal of Gerontology, 37, 91-99.

Pawlarczk, D., & Schumacher, K. (1983). Concurrent validity of the behavior development survey. American Journal of Mental Deficiency, 87, 619-626.

Research Group at Lanterman General Hospital. (1979). Behavior development survey user's manual, individualized data base. Los Angeles: University of California.

Veit, C.T. & Ware, J.E. Jr. (1983). The structure of psychological well-being in general populations. Journal of Consulting and Clinical Psychology, 51, 730-742.

BOOK REVIEWS

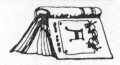

INTEGRATION OF DEVELOPMENTALLY DISABLED INDI-
VIDUALS INTO THE COMMUNITY. Laird W. Heal, Janell I.
Haney, and Angela Novak Amado (Eds.) *2nd Ed. Baltimore, MD:
Paul H. Brookes Publishing Co., 1988, 347 pages, $24.95.*

The twenty-three contributors to this book are authorities in the
fields of education and social science relating to the integration of
the developmentally disabled individual into the community. Therapists serving this population will find much of interest in this in-
depth study.

The purpose of the book, as indicated in the preface, is to summarize the scholastic effort that has been devoted to integrating developmentally disabled citizens into the mainstream of American
life. The preface includes a brief overview of each chapter. There
are helpful summaries at the end of the chapters.

The authors present the history of community integration from its
beginnings, examining the positive aspects and presenting the concerns which have arisen. Although many problems remain to be
solved, one author held the viewpoint that with adequate support
services any client could succeed in his or her residential arrangement.

Chapter 8, on training in community and living skills, is of particular interest to occupational therapists. It states clearly that successful community living is associated with the ability to use daily
living skills. The opinion expressed that critical skills must be
taught in elementary school years with family cooperation is shared

by occupational therapists in the field. The author indicates generalization of skills and long time behavior maintenance are areas needing research and program development.

Chapter 10, on meaningful employment outcomes, is an excellent resource for therapists in vocational situations dealing with the developmentally disabled population. The author reviews the history of work-related programming from 1966 when the Fair Labor Standards Act authorized the establishment of work activity centers to serve persons unable to benefit from preparation for competitive employment. Various methods of work-related training are analyzed and discussed. The current Supported Employment model is presented positively along with obstacles to successful competitive employment. He concludes that meaningful employment provides persons with severe disabilities the greatest opportunity to interact with non-disabled peers in a normalized work environment.

As supplementary reading, I suggest therapists involved in helping adults with developmental disabilities read Lana Warren's article titled, *Helping the Developmentally Disabled Adult* (1986) *American Journal of Occupational Therapy*, 40, page 227. She directs our attention to the great need which exists for therapists to choose to work with adults with developmental disabilities. She stresses their need for our focus on purposeful activity with orientation toward self maintenance, work, and play/leisure which clearly relates us to this group.

Jane T. Herrick, OTR

LIVING SKILLS FOR MENTALLY HANDICAPPED PEOPLE.
Christine Peck and Chia Swee Hong. *London and Sydney: Croom Helm Ltd, Provident House, 1988, 221 pages.*

The goal of the authors is to unite theory and practice for the benefit of therapists and others entering the field of independence for persons with multiple handicaps. They initially discuss the importance of multi-disciplinary teamwork, and examine normalization in a thorough, challenging manner.

Their approach to programming for new skills or desired behavior changes presents specific intervention techniques that are analyzed clearly and easily understood. Readers will appreciate the frequent examples of successful techniques and the explanation of when and why some may be contra-indicated.

The reason for and requirements of effective assessment are detailed in an informative manner. Definitions of the various types of assessments are given, and the selected listing offers a quick look at the wide range of current tests available for the ongoing process of meeting client needs. This is followed by a chapter that clearly describes the procedure for writing treatment programs, and shows sample teaching charts that make training consistent.

The book deals in depth with the concepts of basic, intermediate and advanced living skills. Each level is introduced by covering its characteristic physical, sensory and perceptual abilities, then giving many practical training suggestions. Planning for group sessions with related therapeutic activities is presented in detail. There are well-structured examples of appropriate media, each outlining objectives, equipment and methods.

For anyone involved in training people with disabilities to become less dependent, this is an exciting text. It is instructive and useful for practical application. The authors, both occupational therapists, have achieved their goal and furnished a very valuable resource that encourages quality programming.

Helen E. Lowe, OTR

THE COGNITIVE REHABILITATION WORKBOOK: A SYSTEMATIC APPROACH TO IMPROVING INDEPENDENT LIVING SKILLS IN BRAIN INJURED ADULTS. Pamela M. Dougherty and Mary Vining Radomski. *Rockville, MD: Aspen Publishers, Inc., 1987, 299 pages, $48.00.*

This Workbook was designed by two occupational therapists as a treatment tool for use with high functioning head-injured adults during the final phase of the rehabilitation process. The authors state that it may also have application to other diagnoses such as stroke, mental illness or mental retardation.

The Workbook can be used in treatment settings to teach cognitively impaired individuals to improve their own basic living skills by providing activities that promote self-awareness, independence and compensatory strategies for permanent higher level cerebral deficits. Graded activities are provided which relate to daily living and work behaviors. The goal is to build the necessary skills for independent living and successful reentry into the workplace.

The Workbook is divided into four major sections. Section I provides an overview of cognitive rehabilitation, a description of the Workbook, and how to use the activities in cognitive rehabilitation treatment sessions. A case study is provided to demonstrate application with an actual patient. This is very helpful in providing a clear picture of how one might use and adapt the activities provided and how long it might take a patient to achieve desired results.

Section II provides a pre- and post-assessment of work related behaviors. Designed as an adjunct to the information therapists would have reviewed from other sources, this assessment helps to determine whether the activities in the Workbook could benefit the patient and the patient's readiness to begin treatment at a specific cognitive level.

Section III includes information for training a patient to develop and use a memory notebook. This is designed to become a true "memory prosthesis." A step-by-step approach is presented to train the patient in successful development of a practical guide for remembering daily activities.

Section IV contains nine training units in the areas of comprehension, computations, managing a checking account, meal planning, giving and receiving directions, using resources such as the telephone, understanding and maintaining schedules and calendars, locating necessary information within newspapers, and personal time management. Each unit contains graded activities divided into three levels of difficulty which are color coded red (easiest), white and blue (hardest). The patient and therapist mutually agree upon goals for each activity. The activities can thus be tailored to a patient's specific needs. Each unit also contains a personal application task which is designed to coincide with a specific need in the patient's current life situation.

The Workbook contains all the forms, score sheets, and instructions needed to complete each activity in a three ring binder format. It is designed to be used individually. However, the authors state that some of the activities might be done in group settings, as well.

The Workbook provides a useful resource for therapists treating patients in the final stages of cognitive rehabilitation. It addresses treatment needs in an area in which remaining deficits often limit the patient from achieving his/her maximum potential level of recovery. The authors acknowledge that the data obtained from these treatment activities have not been published. However, their aim is to share an approach which has been successful for them over a five year period and to provide a time-saving resource to others who are working with this population.

Anne B. Blakeney, OTR

BRAIN INJURY REHABILITATION: A NEUROBEHAVIORAL APPROACH. Rodger L. Wood. *Rockville, MD: Aspen Publishers, Inc., 1987, 196 pages.*

This is a detailed and extensively researched book covering both theoretical and clinical implications of a neuropsychological approach to treatment of brain injury. It is of value to clinicians working in structured brain injury units or those involved in program design of such units. While this approach has been described before, this book is unique in documenting its success with severely brain injured patients an average of five years post trauma.

The book begins with an examination of problem behaviors of brain injured people. Dr. Wood points out that problems of behavior are often more critical than physical deficits in preventing patients from returning to their families and communities. Generalized rehabilitation centers are often poorly equipped to treat behavior problems, especially poor motivation and threatening or embarrassing behaviors. If these behaviors go untreated they often interfere with the patient's ability to benefit from physical rehabilitation. This has become well accepted, as is seen by the proliferation of specialized brain injury units in rehab centers and centers which treat only brain injury.

The neurobehavioral approach described by Dr. Wood involves first analyzing the behavior, describing it accurately and determining whether it relates to events in the person's life or environment. Behaviors which occur with no relationship to environmental events need to be treated medically. Other behaviors are treated via operant conditioning. Organically determined behavior disorders described include aggression, disinhibited behaviors and disorders of arousal, motivation and responsiveness. While these behaviors may be organic in origin, parts of them may be learned. Premorbid personality is often a factor, and disruptive behaviors are often rewarded by attention from busy hospital personnel, especially in early stages of injury.

The treatment described by Dr. Wood took place in the Kemsley Unit of St. Andrew's Hospital Northampton, for several years beginning in 1979. The Unit was "designed as a specialised rehabilitation unit for patients with post traumatic behavior disorders, severe enough to prevent rehabilitation taking place in conventional units or the person being accepted back into the community" (pp. 41-42). Treatment included all rehabilitation therapies provided in a token economy system designed to reinforce specific behaviors. Tokens could be used to obtain rewards and privileges such as meals, cigarettes, use of TV, visits to relatives and movies. Praise and encouragement were also used as positive reinforcement. Negative punishment was utilized in the form of time outs, including use of a locked time-out room for patients showing physical aggression. Positive punishment took the form of aromatic ammonia vapor held under the patient's nose following a specific undesirable behavior.

Dr. Wood uses the single case study design to evaluate the efficacy of treatment at Kemslcy, and devotes a full chapter to discussion of statistical methods and design, including the limitations of the method. The remainder of the book presents numerous case studies describing the results of the various forms of neuropsychological treatment on different behavior disorders, including aggression, inappropriate sexual behaviors and habits. Behavioral techniques were also applied to rehabilitation therapies including physiotherapy, speech therapy and ADL training. Of special interest to occupational therapists are several cases describing how the token economy was used to improve self care skills, and how treatment was broken down into simple units that took into account patients' cognitive deficits.

While Dr. Wood accomplishes his goal of showing the statistical efficacy of the treatment methods he uses, I would have liked to learn more about the long term effect of treatment and the effect of return to community or other settings on the patients and their new behaviors. This is a solid addition to the literature on neurobehavioral treatment. It is a scholarly work and does not make for easy reading, but it provides the interested reader with valuable information on neurobehavioral treatment of severely brain injured patients.

Judith Dicker, OTR

SPLINTING THE BURN PATIENT. Carol Walters. *Laurel, MD:RAMSCO Publishing Company, 1987, 97 pages.*

In her introduction, the author states that *Splinting the Burn Patient* was written to aide therapists who are unfamiliar or who have limited experience with burn splinting. The book succeeds in meeting this objective and provides the novice burn therapist with basic splinting information and guidelines.

Splinting the Burn Patient is divided into twelve chapters. The first two chapters review basic splinting techniques and pattern making. Although basic, the information presented on splinting techniques is clearly written and practical. The splinting material used in this book is limited to polyform. Information on the use of alternative plastics for splinting is not provided. The author has extensive experience in splinting with polyform and provides the reader with tips that will help the novice use polyform more efficiently.

The remaining ten chapters are divided anatomically into parts of the body such as the face, neck, axilla, elbow, hand, knee and foot. Specific chapters are presented on the wrist, hand, palm, and thumb web space. The divisions are logical and easy to follow. Splinting techniques are clear, but protocols related to philosophy and use are brief. Therapists who are in need of a comprehensive primer on splinting the burn patient will find more specific information in Maude Malick's *Splinting Handbook for Burns.*

The photographs used in the book are useful and informative but are amateur in quality. Photographs of complex splints using intricate strapping patterns are sometimes confusing due to the use of excessive labeling and limited sequential step-by-step detailed instructions. The inexperienced therapist may have some difficulty following the directions provided for the more difficult splints and straps such as those for the thumb web space, axilla and elbow.

While providing practical instructions, the author does not include any resources or a recommended reading list. The book is addressed to the clinician rather than to the theorist or researcher.

Splinting the Burn Patient is a good, basic introductory manual to splinting techniques useful with burns. It can serve as a valuable resource for therapists who have had limited experience working with the burn patient. The "cookbook" approach used by the author is practical and easily integrated into the clinical setting. It is highly recommended as a basic resource manual for the therapist with little or no burn experience.

Cynthia Burt, OTR

INTRODUCTION TO RESEARCH: A GUIDE FOR THE HEALTH SCIENCE PROFESSIONAL. Carol K. Oyster, William P. Hanten, and Lela A. Llorens. *Philadelphia, PA: J. B. Lippincott Co., 1988, 239 pages, $16.95.*

Introduction to Research: A Guide for the Health Science Professional is intended to be an introductory methods text for the novice researcher or consumer of research. In the first chapter, Oyster, Hanten and Llorens state that their mission in writing this book is to improve the reputation of the health professions as bonafide sciences by promoting empirical investigation as the dominant epistemology. The remainder of Chapter One provides basic introductory guidelines for selecting a research question, conducting a literature review and evaluating research articles. Practical skills such as efficient use of the library are included in this section. The organization of the book then follows the sequence of the empirical, deductive research process.

Chapter Two is entitled Stating the Problem. The reader is familiarized with the role of theory as the basis for the selection of a research problem and for the structure of the investigative strategy. Levels of abstraction are then organized into a model of scientific development, following which basic terminology is introduced and defined.

An extensive discussion of validity, reliability and sampling is presented to the reader in Chapter Three. The authors have based their discussion of these fundamental concepts on widely used and accepted works such as those of Cook and Campbell, thereby creating a strong chapter for the knowledgeable researcher. However, for the novice, this chapter may prove to be somewhat confusing due to its complexity and to the use of terms (i.e., parametric and nonparametric) which have not been previously defined in the text.

Chapters Four, Five and Six guide the reader through three basic categories of research design: Pre-experimental and Experimental; Quasi-Experimental and Non-experimental. Each design is described and analyzed for its usefulness and rigor. The degree of control, manipulation of variables and potential for randomization are considered as the indicators of desirability for each design.

Data collection techniques logically follow the discussion of design. In Chapters Seven and Eight, the reader is familiarized with methods by which data are obtained and organized for analysis. Chapter Eight includes a particularly useful section on instrument construction.

Before statistics are introduced, the authors have included a summary chapter, Chapter Nine, in which experimental bias and some superficial ethical considerations are addressed.

The Chapters on data analysis are, in the opinion of this reviewer, the strongest section of this text. Statistics are presented to the novice in a simplified fashion. The omission of the computational aspect of data analysis gives the reader the opportunity to develop a conceptual understanding of the application of various statistical procedures to data analysis without intimidation.

The remaining two chapters focus on practical issues of research such as use of the computer and guidelines for reporting research.

While many sections are well written and potentially useful to the researcher who is beginning to explore empirical methodology, this text may have limited use for health professionals who are interested in research. Firstly, there is an inconsistent level of difficulty throughout the text. While some chapters are aimed specifically at the novice, such as those dealing with use of the library and writing a research report, other sections (i.e., those on validity and reliability) require that the reader have prerequisite knowledge of empirical epistemology before concepts may be fully understood.

Secondly, and most importantly, the ideological underpinnings of this text may be inconsistent with emerging research trends and needs within the health professions. In the opinion of this reviewer, while there is a fundamental place for scientific method in the health sciences, the strict adherence to positivistic methodology promoted by this book may be in conflict with the level of theory development and the nature of the research questions in the health professionals. If, as the authors state, the purpose of research is to generate knowledge, this text misses the mark. Scientific information is only one aspect of knowledge and is not sufficient to explain the complex phenomena of human health and methods by which health can be promoted by the health professions. To lead the reader to believe that research which does not employ true experimental design is inferior seems to be a disservice to the researcher as well as to the health professions. It is this reviewer's opinion that an introductory research text must include an overview of the spectrum and application of empirical and normative approaches to knowledge generation, and provide the reader with the understanding that the way in which research questions are posed and answered will determine the knowledge which emerges from the research effort.

Elizabeth DePoy, OTR

SPINAL CORD INJURY: A GUIDE TO FUNCTIONAL OUTCOMES IN OCCUPATIONAL THERAPY. S. Intagliata, Occupational Therapy Series Editor. *Rockville, MD: Aspen Publishers, Inc., 1986, 237 pages, $44.50.*

This book is one in a series of publications from the Rehabilitation Institute of Chicago (RIC) and the first volume in a series to be completed by the Occupational Therapy Department.

As stated in the preface, this book grew out of a need to develop uniform standards of clinical care which could be used to monitor the appropriateness and effectiveness of occupational therapy treatment at RIC. The format focuses on the identification of behavioral indicators in the recovery process and defines and describes concepts, evaluation protocols and relevant treatment planning.

The reader will find units on evaluation, goal setting, treatment planning, strengthening activities, deformity control, a variety of self care and hygiene activities, and discharge planning. Appendices at the end list sources of equipment presented in the book as well as a reference and reading list.

At the beginning of each unit, the authors provide the theory of and present the rationale for recommendations on the specific topic being addressed. Included in each unit is a "Summary Chart" which lists goals, physical indicators for each goal and recommended intervention. These summaries are a bit difficult to interpret initially but once the reader becomes familiar with the format, they provide a quick reference to treatment. One chart with which this reviewer had a particularly difficult time was the "Activities of Daily Living Chart." There is no key on the chart itself, thus, the reader must refer back to the abbreviations in the Introduction to interpret the information.

Therapists and students unfamiliar with balanced forearm orthoses (BFO'S) will find the table in the unit on deformity control particularly useful. It contains a table which identifies BFO parts, lists the motions facilitated by each part, presents the mechanism to accomplish the motion and provides the functional implications.

Perhaps one of the most valuable contributions this book makes is the many photographic illustrations. Treatment techniques, orthotic equipment, self care techniques and equipment are clearly presented so they can be easily duplicated.

Students and entry level therapists working with spinal cord injured persons will find this book an invaluable addition to their list of resources. Experienced therapists may find it a useful means of refreshing their memory and making sure all areas of treatment have been considered. There is, however, little new information for therapists experienced in the treatment of spinal cord injury.

Mary W. McKenzie, MSED, OTR, FAOYA